Statistics for Biomedical Engineers and Scientists

Statistics for Biomedical Engineers and Scientists

How to Visualize and Analyze Data

Andrew P. King

Robert J. Eckersley

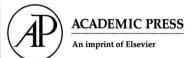

ACADEMIC PRESS
An imprint of Elsevier

Academic Press is an imprint of Elsevier
125 London Wall, London EC2Y 5AS, United Kingdom
525 B Street, Suite 1650, San Diego, CA 92101, United States
50 Hampshire Street, 5th Floor, Cambridge, MA 02139, United States
The Boulevard, Langford Lane, Kidlington, Oxford OX5 1GB, United Kingdom

Library of Congress Cataloging-in-Publication Data
A catalog record for this book is available from the Library of Congress

British Library Cataloguing-in-Publication Data
A catalogue record for this book is available from the British Library

ISBN: 978-0-08-102939-8

For information on all Academic Press publications
visit our website at https://www.elsevier.com/books-and-journals

Working together
to grow libraries in
developing countries

www.elsevier.com • www.bookaid.org

Publisher: Mara Conner
Acquisition Editor: Tim Pitts
Editorial Project Manager: Joshua Mearns
Production Project Manager: Kamesh Ramajogi
Designer: Mark Rogers

Typeset by VTeX

Dedication

A.P.K. – *For my parents, Bernard and Maureen.*

R.J.E. – *In memory of Prof. David Cosgrove.*

"*The quiet statisticians have changed the world, not by discovering new facts or technical developments but by changing the ways we reason, experiment, and form our opinions about it.*"

Ian Hacking

Contents

About the Authors

Andrew King has over 15 years of experience of teaching courses at university level. He is currently a Reader in Medical Image Analysis in the School of Biomedical Engineering and Imaging Sciences at King's College London.

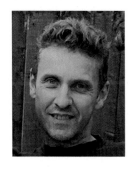

In 2001–2005, Andrew worked as an Assistant Professor in the Computer Science department at Mekelle University in Ethiopia and was responsible for curriculum development, design, and delivery of modules.

Andrew's research interests focus on the use of machine learning and medical imaging to learn clinically useful information, with a special emphasis on moving organs (http://kclmmag.org).

Robert Eckersley has been a Senior Lecturer in the School of Biomedical Engineering and Imaging Sciences at King's College London since 2012. He has been teaching at undergraduate and postgraduate levels since 2006. Prior to 2012, Robert was a lecturer in the Department of Imaging Sciences at Imperial College London.

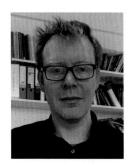

Robert's research is centered around the use of ultrasound in medical imaging. He has a long standing interest in the use of microbubbles as contrast agents for ultrasound imaging.

Together Andrew and Robert run the Computational Statistics module for Biomedical Engineering students upon which this book was based.

Preface

AIMS AND MOTIVATION

Recent years have seen a rapid increase in the use of technology in healthcare, and the field of statistics provides essential tools for understanding and testing the impact of new biomedical technologies and techniques. The authors have been teaching an undergraduate module on statistics using MATLAB® for Biomedical Engineering students at King's College London for a number of years, and this book has grown out of this experience. We have seen the wide range of challenges, difficulties, and misconceptions faced by students when trying to learn about statistical techniques and their practical application in biomedicine, and we have developed a variety of ways of addressing them. We have tried to incorporate these into this book, and we hope that the result is a clear and logically structured introduction to the fundamental concepts of statistics, featuring intuitive explanations motivated by realistic examples.

The module that we have been teaching is aimed at Biomedical Engineering students, and so most of the examples and exercises reflect this fact. However, we believe that the content of the book and its presentation will be more widely applicable. Therefore the intended audience of this book is any undergraduate or postgraduate student who wants to learn the fundamentals of visualizing and analyzing data using statistical techniques. We also believe that researchers working in the biomedical sciences and related areas who are looking to include statistical analysis in their work may benefit from the book.

We believe that it is important not just to learn *how* to apply statistical methods, but also to appreciate some of their underlying concepts and theory. The content of this book reflects this belief. However, we stop short of including lengthy mathematical proofs and derivations of the techniques we present, but rather we try to get across an "intuitive" feel for the underlying theory. To make things easier for the reader, we often separate these explanations of *why* techniques work from the descriptions of *how* they can be applied. This allows the readers to have more flexibility in how they use the book. If you are only interested in quickly getting started on using statistics to analyze and visualize your data, then you can skip these sections (which are boxed off with the heading *The Intuition*). If, however, you want to come to a deeper understanding of the methods that you are using (which we hope you do), then you can read and understand these extra sections.

At the beginning of each chapter, clear learning objectives are provided. In the chapter bodies a range of practical biomedical examples are used to illustrate the concepts being presented. We also include *Activities* in the chapter bodies, which enable the reader to test how well they have met each of the learning objectives. Solutions to all activities are available from the book's web site. We use MATLAB to illustrate the practical application of the statistical techniques we describe.[1] However, the MATLAB content is included at the *end* of each chapter in a separate section, which can then be used by the reader to solve the practical *Exercises* that follow (which are also linked to the learning objectives at the beginning of the chapter). Therefore it is possible to read this book purely as a book about statistics and not engage with the MATLAB content at all. Having said this, using an automated tool such as MATLAB makes visualizing and analyzing data a lot easier, so we strongly recommend using one, even if it is not MATLAB. We have done our best to ensure the realism of the data that we use in our examples, activities, and exercises, and which are freely accessible to the reader on the book's web site. However, all data are completely synthetic, and we take full responsibility for any lack of realism.

At the end of each chapter, we include a brief pen portrait of a famous figure from the history of the field of statistics. Statistics is sometimes viewed as a dry and lifeless subject. We hope that by bringing to life some of these significant figures and linking their work to the concepts that we present, we can help to overcome this myth.

Learning Objectives

On completion of the book the reader should be able to:

- Demonstrate an understanding of the fundamental concepts of descriptive and inferential statistics.
- Analyze data and choose an appropriate hypothesis test to answer a given question.
- Compute numerical statistical measures and perform hypothesis tests "by hand".
- Visualize data and perform statistical analysis using MATLAB.
- Analyze a problem and design an experiment to gather the required data to answer questions about it.

---

[1] All MATLAB codes are compatible with version 2018a.

HOW TO USE THIS BOOK

Instructors

It is our intention that the book can be easily used as a companion to a taught undergraduate or postgraduate module on statistics. We provide a full set of teaching materials to instructors, which they are free to make use of and modify as they see fit. The book consists of eleven chapters, each of which could reasonably be covered in a week of teaching. Depending on how many weeks are available, instructors can use all or a selection of the chapters.

In our module at King's College London we perform all teaching in a computer laboratory. This allows us to quickly link theoretical concepts to practical application and encourages hands-on skill acquisition. The teaching materials are based upon this approach. However, if instructors prefer to separate the theory and applications, for example, by having dedicated lectures and practical laboratory sessions, then the materials can be adapted accordingly.

We recommend that the learning objectives included at the beginning of each chapter should be used as the basis for any assessments. For example, a written exam could test knowledge of the non-MATLAB learning objectives, and/or practical courseworks could be used to test the MATLAB learning objectives.

Students and Researchers

The book can also be used as a stand-alone teaching resource for the interested reader. Our recommended approach in this case is to work through the book chapter-by-chapter and attempt all activities to check your progress against the provided learning objectives. If you find any activity difficult, then revisit the corresponding content and review the activity. Once you are confident in your knowledge of the statistical concepts in each chapter, then read the MATLAB implementation section at the end and practice using the provided code and functions on some simple data of your own. Then you can attempt the exercises at the end of each chapter and again assess your progress against the learning objectives. Only when you are sure that you have met all learning objectives, should you move on to the next chapter. Through this approach we believe that you will gain a thorough understanding of the fundamentals of statistical data visualization and analysis and be able to apply it to real-world problems and data of your own.

Web Site Resources

The book comes with companion web-based materials. There are two sets of resources: one for students using the book as a learning aid and one for instructors who wish to base a taught module upon it. The URLs of the sites are:

- *Student site*: https://www.elsevier.com/books-and-journals/book-companion/9780081029398. This site is freely available to all and contains many code examples and all data required to attempt the MATLAB exercises at the end of each chapter. Solutions to all activities and exercises are also provided.
- *Instructor site*: https://textbooks.elsevier.com/web/Manuals.aspx?isbn=9780081029398. This site is restricted to registered instructors and contains a set of teaching materials that can be used and modified as instructors see fit.

CONTENTS AND ORGANIZATION

The book consists of 11 chapters:

- *Chapter 1 – Descriptive Statistics I: Univariate Statistics*. This chapter provides a general introduction to the field of statistics. The difference between *descriptive* and *inferential* statistics is outlined, and some fundamental concepts and notation regarding the type of data being analyzed are presented. After these introductory concepts the chapter focuses on descriptive statistics of *univariate* data or data in which a single value or variable is measured from each 'individual'.
- *Chapter 2 – Descriptive Statistics II: Bivariate and Multivariate Statistics*. This chapter extends the concepts of the previous chapter to cover descriptive statistics of *bivariate* data or data in which *two* variables are measured per individual. As well as bivariate data visualization techniques, we look at numerical measures of the *correlation* between two variables, the *covariance* between multiple variables, and the use of *Bland–Altman analysis*.
- *Chapter 3 – Descriptive Statistics III: ROC Analysis*. This chapter continues the discussion of descriptive statistical techniques by introducing the concept of *ROC analysis*. ROC analysis is a way of visualizing the performance of a test by comparing its decisions with a known *gold standard*. It builds upon the concepts of *sensitivity* and *specificity* and enables the production of a plot that illustrates how the test performs for a range of different thresholds.
- *Chapter 4 – Inferential Statistics I: Basic Concepts*. After covering descriptive statistics for the first three chapters, this chapter and the next four cover *inferential* statistics. The chapter starts by reviewing the fundamental concepts of probability, which underpin the field of inferential statistics. The key piece of theory presented in this chapter is the *central limit theorem*. The implications of this theorem for inferential statistics are discussed, and based upon this two measures of reliability for estimates of central tendency are introduced, the *standard error of the mean* and *confidence intervals of the mean*.
- *Chapter 5 – Inferential Statistics II: Parametric Hypothesis Testing*. This chapter builds on the basic concepts introduced in Chapter 4 to explain how

hypotheses about data can be formally tested. In particular, the chapter deals with *parametric* hypothesis tests, which typically assume that the data being tested are normally distributed. The *Student's t-test* is introduced as the most common parametric hypothesis test.

- *Chapter 6 – Inferential Statistics III: Nonparametric Hypothesis Testing.* Following on from the treatment of parametric hypothesis testing, this chapter discusses the corresponding *nonparametric* hypothesis tests that can be used when we cannot assume a normal distribution in our data.

- *Chapter 7 – Inferential Statistics IV: Choosing a Hypothesis Test.* To choose an appropriate hypothesis test (i.e. parametric or nonparametric), we must be able to decide whether data fit sufficiently well to a normal distribution. This chapter introduces a range of visual and numerical techniques that can be used to help to make this decision.

- *Chapter 8 – Inferential Statistics V: Multiple and Multivariate Hypothesis Testing.* The preceding chapters on inferential statistics all assume that the data are *univariate* (i.e. one value per 'individual') and that we are only testing a single hypothesis about the data. This chapter introduces some parametric hypothesis tests that can be used when we have data that are *multivariate* (more than one value per 'individual') and/or we want to ask multiple questions about our data.

- *Chapter 9 – Experimental Design and Sample Size Calculations.* Until this point in the book, we have assumed that the data to be visualized and analyzed have already been gathered. This chapter deals with the important topic of how best to design an experiment to gather the right data and to be able to ask and answer questions about it. We discuss the types of errors that can be present in measured data and introduce ways in which experiments can be designed to minimize the effects of these errors. We also explain the principles behind power and sample size calculations.

- *Chapter 10 – Statistical Shape Models.* This chapter introduces the concept of a *statistical shape model* (SSM). SSMs have been hugely influential in the biomedical sciences and have found application in a wide range of areas. They can be viewed as extending the concept of inferential statistics to *shapes* rather than just variables. We cover the theory behind SSMs and how they are closely linked to the concept of *dimensionality reduction*.

- *Chapter 11 – MATLAB Case Study on Descriptive and Inferential Statistics.* The book closes with a realistic biomedical case study to illustrate the use of some of the techniques that have been presented in the preceding chapters. This is the only chapter that involves use of MATLAB throughout, so if you are reading the book purely as a book about statistics and do not care about the use of MATLAB, you can skip this chapter.

Acknowledgments

Above all, we would like to express our gratitude to Graeme Penney. Graeme codeveloped the materials for the original module from which this book was developed. Much of the material in the book is based on Graeme's original notes, and he also wrote early versions of some of the text. We are grateful for Graeme's permission to build on this material to produce this book.

We would like to thank Esther Puyol Antón for providing the MR data that was used in Chapters 10 and 11, and Kawal Rhode for permission to use the image in Fig. 10.3. We also thank all previous King's College London Biomedical Engineering students and teaching assistants on the Computational Statistics module for providing useful and constructive feedback, which has helped to shape the book.

Finally, from the publishers Elsevier we thank Tim Pitts for his encouragement and honest feedback on our original proposal and Joshua Mearns for his assistance during the development of the book.

CHAPTER 1

Descriptive Statistics I: Univariate Statistics

LEARNING OBJECTIVES

At the end of this chapter you should be able to:

O1.A *Explain the reasons for using statistics*
O1.B *Identify different data types*
O1.C *Display univariate statistics in MATLAB*
O1.D *Calculate measures of central tendency (mean, median, mode) by hand and using MATLAB*
O1.E *Calculate measures of variation (standard deviation, interquartile range) by hand and using MATLAB*
O1.F *Decide which statistic and display method is most appropriate for your data*

1.1 INTRODUCTION

We are living in a world in which more and more data are being recorded. As digital and computing advances are made, more data are generated, and more sophisticated machines are developed to allow us to record, track and measure data. Data are recorded in almost every discipline (e.g. economics, health, business, politics, science and engineering), and extremely important decisions are taken based upon analyzing these data. Statistics is the study of how to correctly manipulate data to best inform such decisions. In particular, it helps us to deal with *uncertainty* in measurements. Outside of the world of pure mathematics, data will always contain errors and variation. Statistics enables us to decide when conclusions can be formed, despite our data containing variation. It can be thought of as "mathematics meets the real world."

Statistics can be defined as the *science of collecting and analyzing data*. It can be split into two main categories:

1

Statistics for Biomedical Engineers and Scientists. https://doi.org/10.1016/B978-0-08-102939-8.00010-4

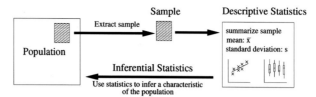

FIGURE 1.1
Overview of how descriptive statistics, inferential statistics, population and sample are related.

- Descriptive Statistics
- Inferential Statistics

The relationship between descriptive and inferential statistics is illustrated in Fig. 1.1. We will use an example problem to help our explanation and introduce a number of statistical terms in *italics* along the way. Imagine that we have been given the task of finding the average height of first-year undergraduate students in the whole country. Height would be termed the *variable* that we aim to measure. The *population* under consideration would be every first-year undergraduate student in the country. To measure and record data from every such student would be very time consuming and costly; therefore we decide just to measure a *sample*, e.g. the height of first-year undergraduate students at a specific college or in a specific class.

Once we have gathered all of the height values from our sample, we need a method to easily make sense of the data. This is the role of *descriptive* statistics, which provides methods to allow us to summarize and describe our sample data. More specifically, descriptive statistics helps us to analyze and understand our results, and to clearly present our results to others.

Inferential statistics is the next stage, in which we attempt to "infer", "deduce", or reach "conclusions" about the population using just information from the sample. This is the subject of Chapters 4–8 of this book. For the next three chapters, we will be concerned with descriptive statistics.

1.2 TYPES OF STATISTICAL DATA

Whether we are using descriptive or inferential statistical techniques, we can always categorize our statistical data into a number of different types. It is important to know what type of data we have as this affects the type of statistical analysis that can be carried out on the data. Carrying out the wrong analysis could lead to incorrect results, or it could mean that we are using our data in a suboptimal way, requiring us to carry out more experiments than necessary. The table below summarizes the four types of statistical data.

Type	Description	Example
Categorical	Variable is non-numerical	Blood type
Ranked	Variable is categorical, where category is an ordered position	Classification of burns (first degree, second degree, etc.)
Discrete	Variable can only take specific values in a given range	Number of blood tests taken
Continuous	Variable can take any value in given range	Blood pressure

Different types of data contain different amounts of information. The amount of information in the data increases from categorical → ranked → discrete → continuous. Categorical variables are just labels and so cannot be ordered in a meaningful way. This limits the type of statistical analysis that can be applied to them. Ranked variables can be ordered, but the distance between values is not meaningful, e.g. is a third degree burn three times as bad as a first degree burn? For discrete and continuous data, the distance between values is meaningful, e.g. the heart of someone with a heart rate of 100 beats per minute (bpm) is beating twice as fast as the heart of someone with a heart rate of 50 bpm. The difference between the discrete and continuous types can sometimes be subtle, e.g. if we measure height to the nearest centimeter, then is this discrete? There is no definite rule for this, but some statisticians use a rule-of-thumb that if a discrete variable can take more than ten values, then it can be treated as continuous.

The number of variables analyzed per "individual" can also vary:

- *Univariate* statistics: A single variable is analyzed.
- *Bivariate* statistics: Two variables per "individual" are analyzed.
- *Multivariate* statistics: Three or more variables per "individual" are analyzed.

This distinction is important to make because the number of variables analyzed also determines the type of analysis that we can perform. In this chapter, we discuss descriptive statistical techniques for *univariate* data, and in the next chapter we deal with bivariate and multivariate descriptive statistics. Chapters 4–6 deal with inferential statistical analysis of *univariate* data, whereas *bivariate* and *multivariate* inferential statistical techniques are discussed in Chapter 8.

■ Activity 1.1

O1.B   For each of the following samples, state what type of data have been collected (i.e. categorical, ranked, discrete or continuous):

1. The *gender* of students in a class.
2. The *height* in millimeters of students in a class.
3. The *number of siblings* (i.e. brothers and/or sisters) for each individual in a class.
4. The *birth order* (i.e. first born, second born) of each individual in a class.
5. The *distance* that each individual in a class travels to get to college.
6. The *type of degree* (e.g. BSc, BEng, BA) that each individual in a class is studying.

■

1.3 UNIVARIATE DATA VISUALIZATION

Descriptive statistics encompasses both visualization techniques, that can help us to better understand the nature of the data that we have acquired and numerical techniques that can enable us to quantitatively summarize the data. We start off with visualization techniques for univariate data.

The simplest way to view data values is to present them in a table. Tables 1.1 and 1.2 show data gathered from 40 first-year undergraduate students: Table 1.1 shows continuous height data, and Table 1.2 shows categorical gender data. The values in the two tables are corresponding; e.g. the first value in each table refers to a male student who is 183 cm tall. Although we can easily see all of the data values, it is not so easy to understand the nature of the data sets as a whole. For example, how many female students are there, or how tall is the tallest student? We are now going to look at some common visual techniques to display these data for easier analysis.

1.3.1 Dotplot

A dotplot, as shown in Fig. 1.2, can provide an initial visual overview of a data set. A dotplot simply plots a single dot for each of the univariate variable values along the x-axis. If multiple identical values occur, then the dots are stacked using the y-axis, as shown by the three counts of 169 shown in Fig. 1.2. Dotplots are most useful for continuous or discrete data in which the distances along the x-axis are meaningful.

A dotplot provides an overview of the entire data set and can be used to obtain an initial impression as to the *distribution* of the data. A statistical *distribution* provides information on the frequency of occurrence of different values. For example, from Fig. 1.2 we can see that no heights greater than 185 cm or less

Table 1.1 Heights of 40 first-year under-graduate students in centimeters.

183	163	152	157	157	165	173	180
164	160	166	157	168	167	156	155
178	169	171	175	169	168	165	166
164	163	161	157	181	163	157	169
177	174	183	181	182	171	184	179

Table 1.2 Genders of 40 first-year under-graduate students: M = Male, F = Female.

M	F	F	F	F	F	M	M
F	F	F	F	F	F	F	F
M	F	F	M	M	F	F	F
F	F	F	F	M	F	F	F
F	F	M	M	M	M	M	M

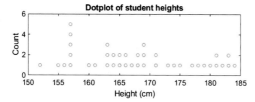

Dotplot of student heights

FIGURE 1.2
Dotplot of first-year undergraduate student heights in cm.

than 150 cm were recorded. Things to look for when assessing a data set using a dotplot include:

- Does the distribution look symmetric?
- Are there any outliers?[1]
- Are the dots evenly distributed, or are there peaks?

1.3.2 Histogram

A similar type of visualization to the dotplot, and one that is more commonly used, is the *histogram*. Histograms are typically used for continuous and discrete data types, and they show the underlying distribution more clearly than

---

[1] *Outliers* are values that are very different to the others in the data set. See Section 1.4.4.

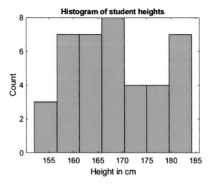

FIGURE 1.3
Histogram of first-year undergraduate student height data.

the dotplot. A histogram of the student height data is shown in Fig. 1.3. As can be seen, it provides a similar visualization to the dotplot, but rather than using stacked dots, it uses bars, whose heights indicate the number of data values in different "bins", or ranges of values. Therefore forming a histogram involves a binning process. Binning describes the process of going from continuous to discrete data (or from discrete data to discrete data with fewer possible values). In Fig. 1.3, seven bins of equal width have been chosen. Every data value should go into one (and only one) bin. Therefore the bins should not overlap and should cover the entire range of the data (i.e. from the lowest to the highest value). It is most common to use bins of equal width. If bins of unequal width are used, then it is important to note that it is the area of the bin that is important, not just the number of counts inside the bin. Therefore, if one bin has twice the width of all the other bins, then the height of that bin should be halved. There are no specific rules on how many bins to use. A rough guide is that the number of bins should be equal to the square root of the number of data values, but not less than six. As is shown in Fig. 1.4, the appearance of a histogram can change depending on the number of bins used. Common sense needs to be applied so that the histogram displays the main features of the data. Also, note that, for large numbers of bins, the histogram is essentially the same as the dotplot.

1.3.3 Bar Chart

For categorical data, and often for ranked data, a bar chart often is an appropriate choice of visualization. Fig. 1.5 shows a bar chart for the categorical gender data from Table 1.2. In a bar chart, distances along the x-axis have no numerical meaning. This is depicted by there being a separation between the columns in the chart (see Fig. 1.5), whereas in a histogram there are no gaps between the columns (see Fig. 1.3).

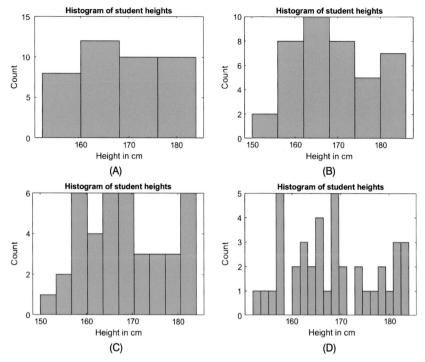

FIGURE 1.4

Histograms of the same student height data with different numbers of bins: (A) 4 bins, (B) 6 bins, (C) 10 bins, (D) 20 bins.

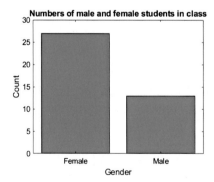

FIGURE 1.5

Bar chart showing numbers of male and female students.

■ **Activity 1.2**

O1.F   Think back to the samples listed in Activity 1.1. For each case, decide how you might best visualize the data.   ■

1.4   MEASURES OF CENTRAL TENDENCY

We now move on from visualization techniques to numerical measures that can be used to quantitatively summarize data. We start off with measures of *central tendency*, which attempt to summarize the "typical" or "average" value in a sample. There are three main measures of central tendency: the *mean*, the *median* and the *mode*. We will first describe the three measures and then discuss the circumstances in which each should be used.

1.4.1   Mean

The mean can be used for continuous or discrete data. It is calculated as

$$\bar{x} = \frac{1}{n} \sum_{i=1}^{n} x_i, \tag{1.1}$$

where:

- ■ x_i represent our individual sample values, e.g. the heights shown in Table 1.1.
- ■ n is the *sample size*, or the number of values we have, e.g. for the data in Table 1.1, $n = 40$.

Note the notation for a mean value, e.g. $\bar{x}$. The bar over a variable name is often used to denote the mean.

1.4.2   Median

The median is the central value of a data set after all of the values have been placed in ascending (or descending) order. Therefore, if there are n values in a data set the median is the $((n+1)/2)$th value. If n is even, then the mean of the two central values is calculated. For example, the median value of our student height sample can be calculated by counting to the $(40+1)/2 = 20.5$th value from either the top or bottom of the dotplot shown in Fig. 1.2. This turns out to be the average of the 20th ($=167$) and 21st ($=168$) values, that is, 167.5 cm. The median is suitable for continuous, discrete or ranked data. It cannot be used for categorical data because, by definition, it is not possible to order the values.

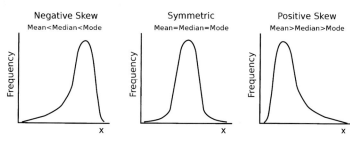

FIGURE 1.6
Example symmetric and skewed distributions.

1.4.3 Mode

The mode simply refers to the most frequently occurring value. This is suitable for all types of data. As an example, the mode of our height data can be seen to be 157 cm, which occurred five times as shown in the dotplot in Fig. 1.2.

1.4.4 Which Measure of Central Tendency to Use?

For continuous or discrete data, the mode is rarely used. Whether to use the mean or median depends upon whether our data distribution is *symmetric* or *skewed,* and whether or not there are *outliers.* Data distributions were discussed earlier in relation to histograms and dotplots. Fig. 1.6 shows examples of symmetric and skewed distributions. Note that the mean, the median and the mode will all have approximately the same value if the data are symmetrically distributed. If the skew is negative (i.e. the left tail of the distribution is longer than the right tail), then the mode will be larger than the median, which in turn will be larger than the mean. The converse is true for positively skewed distributions. Outliers are data points that are very different from the others in the data set being analyzed. It is important to detect them as they may be due to errors in data gathering (e.g. a height entered in meters rather than centimeters). Outliers should not be removed without there being a good reason to do so.

The rules on whether to use mean or median for continuous or discrete data are as follows:

- Use the *mean* if the data distribution is symmetric with no significant outliers.
- Use the *median* if the data distribution is skewed or has significant outliers.

For ranked data, either the median or the mode can be used. Which value to report depends greatly on the data and what we want to show from them.

If the data are categorical, then the choice is easy: we can only calculate the mode.

1.5 MEASURES OF VARIATION

Measures of central tendency only summarize the typical or average value of the data, and they provide no information on its *spread, variation* or *dispersion*. There are two main measures to summarize the spread of data, which are the *standard deviation* and the *interquartile range* (IQR).

1.5.1 Standard Deviation

The sample standard deviation s is defined by

$$s = \sqrt{\frac{1}{(n-1)} \sum_{i=1}^{n} (x_i - \bar{x})^2}, \qquad (1.2)$$

where, as before, n is the sample size, x_i are the individual sample values, and $\bar{x}$ is the sample mean. Note the following points about the standard deviation:

- It has the same units as the data, for example, calculating s for our height data would result in a value in centimeters.
- It is always positive.
- It requires calculation of the mean of the data, $\bar{x}$.
- The division is by $(n-1)$, not n. This makes the value of s a better estimate of the *population* standard deviation.
- The *variance* is the standard deviation squared, that is, s^2.

1.5.2 Interquartile Range

To calculate the interquartile range, we need to calculate the values of the upper and lower *quartiles* of our data. The concept of a quartile is related to the concept of the median, as explained below:

- The *median* is the data value that has 50% of the values above it and 50% of values below.
- The *upper quartile* is the data value that has 25% of values above it and 75% of values below.
- The *lower quartile* is the data value that has 75% of values above it and 25% of values below.

The interquartile range (IQR) is then calculated as

$$\text{IQR} = \text{upper quartile} - \text{lower quartile.} \qquad (1.3)$$

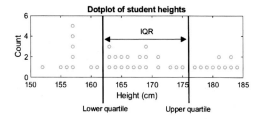

FIGURE 1.7
Values of the IQR and the upper and lower quartile values shown on a dotplot for the first-year undergraduate student height data.

The IQR and upper and lower quartile values for the student height data are shown plotted onto a dotplot in Fig. 1.7. Note that of the 40 data values, 10 are below the lower quartile, 10 are above the upper quartile, and 20 lie within the IQR.

As well as the IQR, the overall *range* of the data is also regularly reported as a measure of variation. The range is simply

$$\text{range} = \text{maximum value} - \text{minimum value}. \tag{1.4}$$

1.5.3   Which Measure of Variation to Use?

The answer to this question is similar to the answer to the question of when to use the mean or median:

- Use the *mean* and *standard deviation* if your data distribution is symmetric with no outliers.
- Use the *median* and *IQR* if your data distribution is skewed or has outliers.

How can we decide if our data distribution is skewed or symmetric? Often it is clear from looking at a histogram, but the following numerical measure can be useful in making this assessment:

$$\text{skew} = \frac{3(\bar{x} - \text{median})}{s}. \tag{1.5}$$

Using this measure, values greater than 1 denote a "reasonable" positive skew, values less than −1 show a "reasonable" negative skew, and values between −1 and 1 show that the distribution is approximately symmetric.

■ **Activity 1.3**

Once more we return to the samples listed in Activity 1.1. This time decide which measures of central tendency and variation should be used to sum-

O1.F

marize these data? Try to consider situations that might alter your initial selection. ■

1.6   VISUALIZING MEASURES OF VARIATION

1.6.1   Visualizing Mean and Standard Deviation

If the mean and standard deviation have been calculated, a standard visualization is to plot the mean value(s) $\bar{x}$ and then to include *error bars*, which show the mean value plus and minus one standard deviation s. Therefore, the error bars are of total length $2 \times s$ and range from $\bar{x} - s$ to $\bar{x} + s$. It is important to state clearly in the caption what the error bars represent, as there are other common uses of error bars such as the *standard error of the mean*, which we will cover in Chapter 4. Fig. 1.8 shows a plot of the mean and standard deviation of the student height data split into male and female data sets.

1.6.2   Visualizing Median and IQR: The Box Plot

If median and IQR have been calculated, then the standard method of visualization is a *box plot* (also known as a *box and whisker plot*), as shown in Fig. 1.9. The meanings of the different parts of the box and whisker plot are labeled in Fig. 1.10. Depending on the software used to produce the plot, outliers are sometimes displayed as individual dots or crosses above or below the "whiskers". In Fig. 1.9, there are no outliers to display.

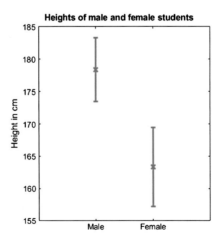

FIGURE 1.8
Plot of mean heights of male and female first-year undergraduate students in centimeters. Error bars denote one standard deviation around the mean.

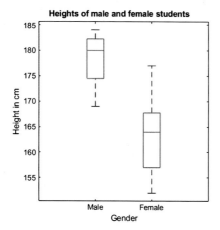

FIGURE 1.9
Boxplots of heights of male and female first-year undergraduate students in centimeters.

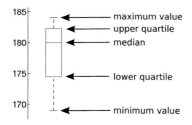

FIGURE 1.10
Values represented by the different parts of a box and whisker plot.

1.7 SUMMARY

Univariate descriptive statistical methods can be used to summarize sample data both visually and numerically. All statistical data can be categorized into one of four different types: categorical, ranked, discrete and continuous. It is important to be able to identify the type of data to know which type of statistical analysis is appropriate. Measures of central tendency (mean, median and mode) provide information on the most "typical" value in a data set. Measures of variation (standard deviation and IQR) provide information on the spread of the data about the "typical" value. If the distribution of the data is symmetric with no significant outliers, then the mean and standard deviation should be used. If the distribution of the data is skewed or has significant outliers, then the median and IQR should be used.

1.8 USING MATLAB FOR UNIVARIATE DESCRIPTIVE STATISTICS

Most of the functions required to perform univariate descriptive statistical analysis are core functions within MATLAB. You can use the MATLAB `doc` or `help` commands to get more information on all of these functions. Where there is no built-in MATLAB function, we provide implementations of our own in the sections below.

Many of the code examples included below make use of the student height data introduced in this chapter. These data are available through the book's web site as "fortyStudentHeightData.mat" and "fortyStudentGenderData.mat". The data are stored as column arrays.

1.8.1 Visualization of Univariate Data

Dotplot:

There is no built-in MATLAB command to produce a dotplot. The function that we provide below, which is available to download as "dotplot.m" from the book's web site, was used to produce the examples in this chapter.

```
function [] = dotplot( x )
% usage:
% [] = dotplot( x )
% x — input list of numbers as column vector
% note no returned values, output is dotplot figure
%
ypos = zeros( length(x), 1 );
for i = 1:length(x)
    for j = i:length(x)
        if  x(j) == x(i)
            ypos(j) = ypos(j) + 1;
        end
    end
end
plot( x, ypos, 'o' );
title('Dotplot');
ylim([0 max(ypos)+1]);
end
```

Histogram:

```
histogram(x,nbins)
```

This produces a histogram from the data in the array x. The parameter `nbins` can be used to specify the number of bins to use in the histogram. If `nbins` is not specified, then MATLAB will automatically determine the number of bins.

Bar Chart:

Bar charts can be produced using the MATLAB `bar` command. The bar chart of student height data shown in Fig. 1.5 was produced using the following code example, which starts from an array of categorical (M or F) values called gender:

```
%load the data
load('fortyStudentGenderData.mat')

%split gender into two separate arrays, one for each gender
male = find(gender=='M');
female = find(gender=='F');

%use the length command to count the number of male and
%female students
%use this as input to the bar plotting function
g = categorical({'Male', 'Female'})
bar(g, [length(male) length(female)]);
title('Numbers of male and female students in class');
xlabel('Gender')
ylabel('Count');
```

Note how the MATLAB `categorical` type is used to set the labels for the bars.

1.8.2   Calculating Measures of Central Tendency

Mean, Median and Mode:

There are built-in commands for each measure of central tendency in MATLAB, as the following code illustrates.

```
load('fortyStudentHeightData.mat');
mean(heights)
%ans = 168.2500
median(heights)
%ans = 167.5000
mode(heights)
%ans = 157
```

1.8.3   Calculating Measures of Variation

Standard Deviation and IQR:

There are built-in commands for each measure of variation in MATLAB, as illustrated in the code below:

```
load('fortyStudentHeightData.mat');
std(heights) %standard deviation
%ans = 9.1083
var(heights) %variance
%ans = 82.9615
```

```
iqr(heights) %inter-quartile range
%ans = 14
range(heights) %range
%ans = 32
```

Upper and Lower Quartiles:

Values for the upper and lower quartiles can be calculated using the `quantile` function. Note that the last parameter denotes which fraction of the data should be below the returned value.

```
load('fortyStudentHeightData.mat');
quantile(heights,0.25) %lower quartile
%ans = 162
quantile(heights,0.75) %upper quartile
%ans = 176
```

Skew:

Using the same data as before, the skew, as defined in Section 1.5.3, can be calculated in MATLAB as follows:

```
3*(mean(heights) - median(heights))/std(heights)
%ans =  0.2470
```

1.8.4   Visualizing Measures of Variation

Error Bars:

The MATLAB `errorbar` function can be used to produce plots with error bars. The following MATLAB commands were used to produce the plot shown in Fig. 1.8:

```
% load data
load('fortyStudentHeightData');
load('fortyStudentGenderData');

% form separate arrays containing male and female height data
maleheight = heights(find(gender=='M'));
femaleheight = heights(find(gender=='F'));

% calculate statistics, and place in arrays
means = [mean(maleheight), mean(femaleheight)];
stdevs = [std(maleheight), std(femaleheight)];

%plot data, and label axes
errorbar(means, stdevs, 'x')
% stop error bar plots from being superimposed on axes
xlim([0 3]);
xticks([1 2]); % set the position of the axis 'ticks'
xticklabels({'Male', 'Female'}); % set tick labels
ylabel('Height in cm')
title('Heights of male and female students');
```

Box Plot:

The MATLAB `boxplot` function produces box plot visualizations. Its first argument is the continuous or discrete data array whose values are to be used for the *y*-axis of the plot. The second argument is a "grouping" variable whose values will be used to split up the data of the first argument. The following MATLAB code was used to produce the box plots shown in Fig. 1.9.

```
% load data
load('fortyStudentHeightData');
load('fortyStudentGenderData');

%the boxplot command can accept a character array as input
%no need to manually sort data
boxplot(heights, gender)
xlim([0 3]);
xticks([1 2]); % set the position of the axis 'ticks'
xticklabels({'Male', 'Female'}); % set tick labels
ylabel('Height in cm')
xlabel('Gender');
title('Heights of male and female students');
```

Note that the default behavior in MATLAB box plots is to consider a data value to be an outlier if it is larger than the upper quartile $+1.5 \times$ IQR or less than the lower quartile $-1.5 \times$ IQR. This is a reasonable way to highlight potential outliers, but it is not a rigorous method to detect them.

1.9 EXERCISES

Perform the following tasks using MATLAB.

■ **Exercise 1.1**

The file "normalBodyTemperature.mat" contains the body temperatures of 130 healthy volunteers in Fahrenheit. Load these data into MATLAB and then carry out the following statistical analysis: *O1.B, O1.C, O1.F*

1. What type of data are we using?
2. Convert the data from Fahrenheit to Celsius:
   $$T_{Celsius} = (T_{Fahrenheit} - 32)/1.8$$
3. Produce a dotplot of the data in Celsius.
4. Visually, is the distribution symmetric or skewed?
5. Visually, are there any outliers?
6. Have a guess at what the medical definition of *hyperthermia* (elevated body temperature) is?
7. Produce a histogram of the Celsius temperature data, with a sensible number of bins.

8. Calculate the most appropriate measure of central tendency (mean, median or mode) to numerically summarize the temperature data in Celsius.

◼

◼ Exercise 1.2

O1.B, O1.C, O1.D,
O1.F

The data in the file "hipImplantNumeric.mat" consist of a numerical code for the types of hip implant used by an orthopaedic surgeon over a one-month period. The numerical code is "Metal–Metal" = 1, "Ceramic–Ceramic" = 2, "Metal–Plastic" = 3, which denotes the composition of the components of the artificial joint.

1. What type of data are we using?
2. Visualize the data using the most appropriate method.
3. Calculate the most appropriate measure of central tendency (mean, median or mode) to summarize the data.

◼

◼ Exercise 1.3

O1.B, O1.C, O1.D,
O1.F

The file "hipImplantNamed.mat" contains the same data as the previous exercise, but the data are stored as implant names rather than using numerical codes. This makes it more difficult to work with the data. In the real world, data rarely arrive in a nice useable format, so it is important to know how to deal with lots of different data types. Repeat the previous exercise using "hipImplantNamed.mat".

The following additional MATLAB commands might be useful to you:

◼ `unique(x)`: Find the unique elements of an array, for example, `typesOfImplant = unique(hipImplantNamed)`
◼ `strcmp(s1,s1)`: Compare the contents of two strings, returning 1 (`true`) if they are identical and 0 (`false`) otherwise, for example, `strcmp('Ceramic–Ceramic', hipImplantNamed)`

◼

◼ Exercise 1.4

O1.B, O1.C, O1.D,
O1.E, O1.F

The data in the file "IGSerrors_mm.mat" consist of absolute error measurements of an image-guided surgery system in millimeters. The required clinical accuracy for the system is 3 mm. Carry out the following statistical analysis on these data:

1. What type of data are we using?
2. Produce a histogram of the data.
3. Calculate the skew of the data using Eq. (1.5).

4. Calculate appropriate numerical measures of central tendency and variation.
5. Display the calculated numerical values using an appropriate plot.
6. Approximately what percentage of accuracy values were below the clinical requirement?

■

■ Exercise 1.5

This exercise uses the same temperature data that were introduced in Exercise 1.1, that is, "normalBodyTemperature.mat". In addition, we will use the file "genderForTemp.mat", which details whether the temperature values in "normalBodyTemperature.mat" were from a male (=1) or female (=2) volunteer. Carry out the following statistical analysis on these data:

O1.B, O1.C, O1.D, O1.E, O1.F

1. What types of data are we using?
2. Convert the temperature data to Celsius.
3. Split the temperature data into separate arrays for male and female volunteers.
4. Analyze the distributions for the male and female temperature data.
5. Calculate appropriate numerical measures of central tendency and variation for the male and female temperature data.
6. Display the calculated numerical values using an appropriate visualization, which should show the male and female data on the same plot.
7. Is there a difference between the male and female temperatures?

■

■ Exercise 1.6

In this exercise, you will generate your own data to investigate whether the mean or the median is the most appropriate measure to use. The MATLAB function randn(m,n) produces an m-by-n matrix of pseudo-random numbers with zero mean and standard deviation 1. The numbers are sampled from a *normal*, or *Gaussian*, distribution. We will discuss the normal distribution in detail in Section 4.4.1, but for now the important information is that the distribution is symmetric with no outliers. Carry out the following investigation:

O1.A

1. Use randn to produce a few 30×1 column vectors of numbers and visualize their distributions by producing histograms. Do they have obvious outliers?
2. Repeat the above (again a few times) but instead of visualizing the data, calculate the mean and median of the numbers. Which of the

measures (mean or median) gives a better estimate of the central value of the distribution (i.e. is closest to the true mean of zero)?

3. Use a loop to repeat the above experiment 100 times. Each time calculate the mean and median values. Use the absolute values of the mean and median (you can use the MATLAB abs function) as error measures. Does the mean or median provide a better estimate of the center of the symmetric distribution?

4. Now repeat the above, but after cubing (i.e. raising to the power of 3) the output from randn. Because we are only using a small sample size (30), this will have the effect of introducing a few outliers. Now see if the mean or median is a better measure to use.

FAMOUS STATISTICIAN: KARL PEARSON

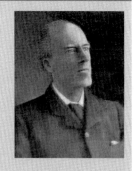

Karl Pearson is one of the most significant figures in the history of statistics and was the inventor of some of the tools still most commonly used by statisticians today. He was born in 1857 in Islington, London, and despite ending up as a famous statistician, in his early life he seemingly had difficulty deciding where his interests lay. He studied subjects as diverse as mathematics, physics, Roman law, medieval German literature and socialism.

He eventually settled upon applied mathematics as his main interest, and perhaps one of his most significant contributions occurred in 1911, when he founded the world's first university statistics department, at University College London. Among his many major contributions to the field are Pearson's r correlation coefficient (see Chapter 2), the foundations of hypothesis testing (see Chapter 5) and the chi-square test (see Chapter 6).

It is perhaps heartening to remember that famous statisticians are humans like the rest of us. One of the themes of Karl Pearson's life and work was the personal enmities he had with two other famous statisticians. He had a long-running and well-known feud with Ronald Fisher, the so-called "Father of Statistics" (see Chapter 8's *Famous Statistician*). In fact, Pearson had actually offered Fisher a job at University College London in 1919, but Fisher turned him down. The personal clash between the two men and the tension between their differing philosophies of statistical analysis represents the deepest rift in the history of the field. However, like Ronald Fisher, Karl Pearson had an active interest in the controversial field of eugenics. Pearson also had a long-running feud with another famous statistician Charles Spearman (see Chapter 2's *Famous Statistician*). Spearman famously criticised Pearson's work in a seminal paper in 1904. Pearson wrote a series of blistering responses to these criticisms, resulting in a bitter and lifelong feud between the two men.

Pearson was a committed socialist and was offered and turned down both an OBE (Order of the British Empire) and a knighthood in his lifetime. He died aged 79 in 1936 in Surrey, UK.

"Statistics is the grammar of science"
Karl Pearson

CHAPTER 2

Descriptive Statistics II: Bivariate and Multivariate Statistics

LEARNING OBJECTIVES

At the end of this chapter you should be able to:

O2.A Choose an appropriate visualization technique for bivariate data and produce a bivariate visualization using MATLAB

O2.B Explain what is represented by a covariance matrix and compute one using MATLAB

O2.C Explain the meaning of Pearson's and Spearman's correlation coefficients, choose an appropriate measure for given data and calculate it using MATLAB

O2.D Calculate the equation of a linear regression line using MATLAB

O2.E Use regression to make estimates by hand and using MATLAB

O2.F Explain and interpret the Bland–Altman plot for investigation of agreement between two measurement methods

O2.G Generate Bland–Altman plots using MATLAB

2.1 INTRODUCTION

In biomedical engineering, we are often interested in how variables relate: for example, how the longevity of a hip implant relates to accuracy of placement, or how brain ventricle size relates to Alzheimer's disease progression. Biomedical engineering experiments are carried out daily by industrial and university research departments to gather data on such relationships. The field of bivariate (and multivariate) descriptive statistics enables us to process such data to help us to understand the relationships between variables and to describe these relationships to others. The statistics that we will cover in this chapter will enable us, amongst other things, to determine the strength of a relationship between variables (*correlation*) and to fit functions to represent the relationship (*regression*). However, it is important to note that the statistical analysis alone will not be able to determine the scientific reason underlying the relationship, and it will not be able to establish *cause-and-effect*, that is, whether manipulating one variable will allow control of the second variable.

Statistics for Biomedical Engineers and Scientists. https://doi.org/10.1016/B978-0-08-102939-8.00011-6

Table 2.1 Degree courses taken by 40 first-year undergraduate students.

BSc	BA	BA	BSc	BSc	BSc	BSc	BSc
BSc	BA	BSc	BA	BSc	BSc	BSc	BA
BSc	BSc	BSc	BSc	BSc	BSc	BSc	BSc
BSc	BSc	BSc	BSc	BSc	BSc	BA	BSc
BA	BSc	BSc	BSc	BSc	BSc	BA	BA

	BSc	BA
M	11	2
F	20	7

FIGURE 2.1
Joint contingency table of student gender and degree type for 40 first-year undergraduate students.

2.2 VISUALIZING BIVARIATE STATISTICS

We start off with visualization techniques. When visualizing two variables at the same time, different visualization methods are possible depending on the types of data involved (i.e. categorical, ranked, discrete, continuous; see Section 1.2). This section introduces some commonly used visualization methods for different combinations of data types. In most cases, categorical and ranked data can be considered to be similar, and discrete and continuous data can be considered together. Therefore in the following examples we only consider two main types, categorical and continuous.

2.2.1 Two Categorical Variables

For two categorical variables, a *joint contingency table* (also often known as a *joint frequency table*) can be a useful way to summarize the data. We will illustrate this using an example in which the two variables are the gender and degree type of a class of 40 undergraduate students. Table 2.1 provides details of whether these students are taking a BA or BSc degree. The genders of the same students were shown in Table 1.2. To summarize these data and to begin to see whether there is a relationship between degree type and gender, we can produce a joint contingency table as shown in Fig. 2.1. The joint contingency table provides a separate row or column for each unique category in the input data. Our example uses a 2 × 2 table because there are two genders (M and F) and two degree types (BA and BSc). The numbers of students with a specific gender who are taking a specific degree type are displayed in the table. These are sometimes presented as percentages. Compared to viewing the original data in Tables 1.2 and 2.1, the summary provided by the joint contingency table enables us, for example, to observe at a glance that a smaller proportion of male students are enrolled on BA degrees.

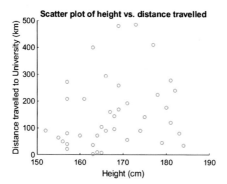

FIGURE 2.2

Scatter plot of student height against distance traveled to university for 40 first-year undergraduate students.

2.2.2 Combining Categorical and Continuous Variables

When we have categorical and continuous data, the basic approach to visualization is to use the categorical data to split up the continuous data into different groups and then to plot these groups' data on the same figure to enable easy comparison. Examples of this were provided in the last chapter when we produced Figs. 1.8 and 1.9, which combined gender (categorical data) with height (continuous data). Recall that, depending on the distribution of the continuous data, we can use either error bars or a box plot to visualize the continuous data for each category.

2.2.3 Two Continuous Variables

The final possibility for bivariate data is when we have two continuous variables. A very useful method to graphically visualize two continuous variables is to produce a *scatter plot*. An example of a scatter plot is shown in Fig. 2.2, in which the student height data used in the previous chapter (Table 1.1) is plotted against the distance each student has had to travel to get to university (data provided in Table 2.2). The scatter plot enables visual inspection of all of the data, and if a relationship between the variables exists, then it can often be clearly seen in a scatter plot. The somewhat random distribution of points in Fig. 2.2 suggests that there is no strong relationship between student height and how far they have traveled.

An alternative to the scatter plot, although not as commonly used, is the 2D histogram. 2D histograms can be created by "binning" the data in the same way as described in the previous chapter for 1D histograms. However, for 2D histograms, bin sizes need to be selected for both variables, and it is not as straightforward to present the number of counts. Figs. 2.3 and 2.4 show two methods for displaying 2D histograms. In Fig. 2.3 the number of counts is

Table 2.2 Distance traveled to university (in km) of 40 first-year undergraduate students.

80	3	90	272	80	8	485	176
10	72	294	22	144	160	50	64
224	480	56	141	259	96	104	90
72	37	208	40	120	400	208	169
410	90	80	278	240	192	35	45

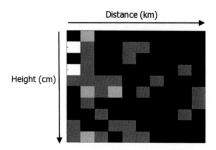

FIGURE 2.3
2D histogram of student height against distance traveled to university. The counts are indicated by image intensities.

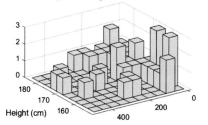

FIGURE 2.4
2D histogram of student height against distance traveled to university. The counts are indicated by the heights of the bars.

presented using image intensity (white = high counts, dark = low counts). In Fig. 2.4 the number of counts is shown using heights in a 3D plot.

On a computer screen the 3D plot in Fig. 2.4 can typically be interactively manipulated and may be a useful way to visualize and examine our data. However, in written reports, 3D plots rarely show information more clearly than well-designed 2D plots.

Finally, line graphs can also be useful for plotting two continuous variables. An example of a line graph is shown in Fig. 2.5. This shows the variation over

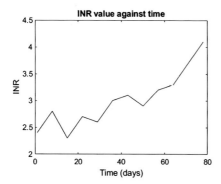

FIGURE 2.5
Line graph of international normalized ratio (INR) against time.

time of a heart patient's *international normalized ratio* (INR). The INR is a ratio derived from a test of blood coagulation, and it is commonly used to adjust the dose of the anticoagulant drug Warfarin. The plot enables easy visualization of how the INR has changed over time.

Generally, line graphs are used in the specific case in which the value of one variable (the *x* variable) can only have a single corresponding value of the other (*y*) variable. Therefore, they are commonly used when one of the variables represents time, as the second variable should only be able to take one value at any given instant in time.

2.2.4 Which Variable Should Go on Which Axis?

A common question to ask when producing plots of two continuous variables is which variable to put on which axis. To answer this question, we need to jump ahead to a topic that we will deal with in detail in Chapter 9: *experimental design*.

There are two main types of experimental design, *experimental* and *observational* studies. Experimental studies produce data in which the researcher is able to alter the value of one variable (often referred to as the *independent variable*) and then measure the value of a second variable (often referred to as the *dependent variable*). An example of this could be altering the pressure applied to an artificial heart valve (pressure is the *independent variable*) and then measuring valve leakage (amount of leakage is the *dependent variable*). When producing figures for data from experimental studies, the independent variable should go on the horizontal axis.

In observational studies, none of the variables are directly altered. An example would be measuring the height and weight of a sample of individuals. Obviously we cannot directly alter either the height or weight – we are just *observing* both of them. When producing figures for data produced from observational

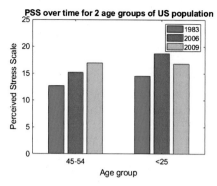

FIGURE 2.6

Bar chart grouped by age group, of Perceived Stress Scale (PSS) for United States' population in three years.

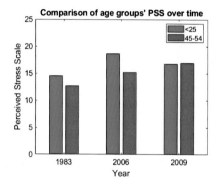

FIGURE 2.7

Bar chart grouped by year, of Perceived Stress Scale (PSS) for two age groups of United States' population.

studies, there are no specific criteria as to which axis should be used for which variable.

2.2.5 General Comments on Choice of Visualization

The choice of visualization method depends greatly upon what is being investigated in the data, or what we wish to show as a main finding in our results. Before displaying data in a report or paper, it is important to logically design the figure so that it most clearly demonstrates the desired relationship. Often, this can be achieved by placing the key values to be compared as close as possible to each other. For example, consider the plots in Figs. 2.6 and 2.7, which visualize data from surveys of *Perceived Stress Scale* within different age groups of the United States' population in three different years [1]. If our primary aim was to investigate whether or not a particular age group had increased their PSS over time, then Fig. 2.6 would be appropriate. However, if, from exactly the same data, the main aim of our investigation was to ascertain in which years one age group had a higher PSS than the other, then Fig. 2.7 would be more appropriate.

■ **Activity 2.1**

Which method of visualization would you use for each of the data sets de-   *O2.A*
scribed below?

1. Favorite food and gender
2. Cholesterol level and time
3. Stride length and age
4. Nationality and height

■

2.3 MEASURES OF VARIATION

2.3.1 Covariance

In Section 1.5.1 the concept of the standard deviation was introduced as a measure of variation for a single continuous or discrete variable. This concept can be extended to the case where we have multiple variables. The corresponding measure of variation for multiple variables (i.e. multivariate data) is known as *covariance*. Covariance is a measure of how much the variations of two variables are related. A positive covariance between two variables reveals that the paired values of both variables tend to increase together. A negative covariance reveals that there is an inverse relationship between the variables, that is, as one increases, the other tends to decrease. A zero covariance indicates that there is no link between the values of the two variables.

For two paired variables x_i and y_i, $i = 1, \ldots, n$ (where n is the sample size), the covariance is defined by

$$cov(x, y) = \frac{1}{n-1} \sum_{i=1}^{n} (x_i - \bar{x})(y_i - \bar{y}). \tag{2.1}$$

Interpretation of the magnitude of the covariance is not straightforward. A quick examination of Eq. (2.1) reveals that the covariance will be larger if the values of the variables themselves are larger. So without some form of normalization it is not possible to use covariance to determine how strong the relationship between the variables is. Pearson's correlation coefficient (see Section 2.4.1) does exactly this by normalizing the covariance by the product of the standard deviations of the variables.

2.3.2 Covariance Matrix

To fully describe the variation of a multivariate data set, we need to compute the covariances between all possible pairs of variables. These values are commonly grouped together and represented as the *covariance matrix*. For example, for two variables x_i and y_i, $i = 1, \ldots, n$ (where n is the sample size), the covariance matrix is defined as

$$C = \begin{pmatrix} cov(x, x) & cov(x, y) \\ cov(y, x) & cov(y, y) \end{pmatrix}. \tag{2.2}$$

Note that the diagonals of C are in fact just the variances of the individual variables as defined in Eq. (1.2), and the other elements of the matrix are the covariance values as defined by Eq. (2.1). Note also that $cov(x, y)$ is the same as $cov(y, x)$ so the covariance matrix is symmetric.

More generally, if we have a sample of *column vectors* $\mathbf{x}_i$ (again $i = 1, \ldots, n$, where n is the sample size), each of which contains the values of multiple variables, the covariance matrix can be defined as

$$C = \frac{1}{n-1} \sum_{i=1}^{n} (\mathbf{x}_i - \bar{\mathbf{x}})(\mathbf{x}_i - \bar{\mathbf{x}})^T. \tag{2.3}$$

Note the similarity between this equation and Eq. (2.1), which defined the covariance between a pair of variables.

2.4 CORRELATION

2.4.1 Pearson's Correlation Coefficient

Pearson's correlation coefficient[1] provides a numerical value that quantifies how linearly related two variables are. As noted before, its formulation is closely linked to that of covariance, as we can see from the following definition:

$$r = \frac{\sum_{i=1}^{n}(x_i - \bar{x})(y_i - \bar{y})}{\sqrt{\sum_{i=1}^{n}(x_i - \bar{x})^2}\sqrt{\sum_{i=1}^{n}(y_i - \bar{y})^2}}, \tag{2.4}$$

where x_i and y_i are the two variables, $i = 1, \ldots, n$, and n is the sample size.

The value of r can range from $+1$ (perfect positive correlation) to -1 (perfect negative correlation). Values of r close to zero suggest no linear correlation. Fig. 2.8 shows example scatter plots and the corresponding values of r. The key points to note from this figure are:

---

[1]This was devised by and named after Karl Pearson; see Chapter 1's *Famous Statistician*.

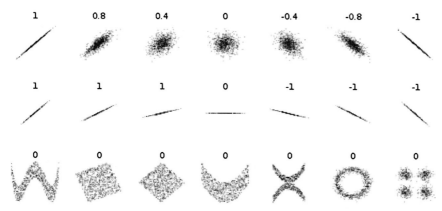

FIGURE 2.8
Example scatter plots and corresponding Pearson's correlation coefficients. Adapted from *http:// en.wikipedia.org/ wiki/ Pearson_product-moment_correlation_coefficient*.

- *Top row*. These plots illustrate how r relates to dispersion from a straight line. The closer the point distribution is to a straight line, the larger is the magnitude of r.
- *Middle row*. The slope of the line does *not* affect the magnitude of r (apart from positive slope $r = +1$, negative slope $r = -1$ and zero slope $r = 0$).
- *Bottom row*. The correlation coefficient only looks for *linear* relationships. Our data may have very strong nonlinear relationships (as shown) and $r = 0$. This emphasizes how important it is to visualize our data (e.g. with a scatter plot) as well as calculate numerical values such as correlation.

Note that a strong correlation between two variables does not signify cause-and-effect. Sometimes correlation occurs simply by chance, that is, there are many variables that can be measured, some of which will increase over time, and some of which will decrease. Just because two variables increase over the same time period (i.e. they are correlated), it does not mean that they are linked in any way at all. For example, between 1996 and 2000 in the United States there was a strong negative correlation ($r = -0.9887$) between highway deaths and lemon imports, as shown in Fig. 2.9. Should the United States' government have restricted lemon imports to make their roads safer?

Correlation can also occur because there is a much stronger third factor influencing both variables. For example, there is a strong correlation between ice cream sales and incidences of drowning. Does ice cream consumption cause drowning? No, both are related by a much stronger third factor, daily temperature. We call this third factor a *confounding variable*.

■ **Activity 2.2**

The following correlations are correct, but are the subsequent deductions valid?   *O2.B*

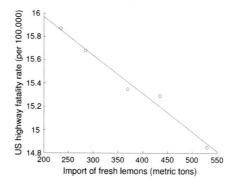

FIGURE 2.9
Scatter plot of US highway deaths against lemon imports over 5 consecutive years 1996 to 2000. The plot shows a strong negative correlation ($r = -0.9887$).

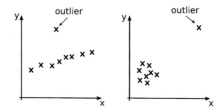

FIGURE 2.10
Examples of how a single outlier can greatly reduce (left) or greatly increase (right) a correlation coefficient value.

1. A child's shoe size is positively correlated with their spelling ability, and therefore large feet should be encouraged to aid literacy.
2. Countries that add chlorine to their water system have a higher incidence of cancer, and therefore chlorine in water causes cancer.

The correlation coefficient can be greatly affected by outliers, as shown in Fig. 2.10. Adding just one extra data point (the outlier) can significantly increase or decrease the correlation coefficient. When faced with such cases, it is important not to simply reject the outlier to get the result that we want. Outliers should only be rejected with good reason. For example, perhaps there was an error in making the measurement?

As an example of the presence of an outlier, consider Table 2.3, which contains data on weekly household expenditure on alcohol and tobacco products in the United Kingdom broken down by geographical region. Fig. 2.11 shows that most of the data appear to show a reasonable linear relationship with a positive slope, but that one data point looks to be an outlier. Calculating the correlation coefficient for all data gives the result $r = 0.22$, which suggests a weak positive correlation. However, after removing the outlier, the remaining

Table 2.3 Weekly household expenditure, in pounds, on alcohol and tobacco products per region (from a British government survey around 1981).		
Region	**Alcohol**	**Tobacco**
North	6.47	4.03
Yorkshire	6.13	3.76
Northeast	6.19	3.77
East Midlands	4.89	3.34
West Midlands	5.63	3.47
East Anglia	4.52	2.92
Southeast	5.89	3.20
Southwest	4.79	2.71
Wales	5.27	3.53
Scotland	6.08	4.51
Northern Ireland	4.02	4.56

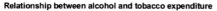

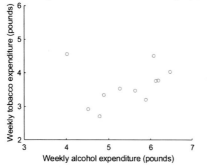

FIGURE 2.11

Scatter plot showing the relationship between weekly household alcohol and tobacco expenditure for different regions of the United Kingdom.

data show a strong correlation (almost 0.8) between weekly tobacco and alcohol expenditure. So a fair summary of the data would be to report both the strong relationship and that one data point appears to be an outlier.

When calculating Pearson's correlation coefficient, it is also possible to derive a *p-value*. In the context of correlation calculations the *p*-value is the probability that the observed relationship between the two variables could have occurred by chance, *assuming that there is actually zero correlation between them*. For example, Fig. 2.12 shows a series of three scatter plots of data consisting of two continuous variables. In each case the values of the first variable were randomly generated, and the values of the second variable were computed by adding a small random offset to the corresponding value of the first variable. In

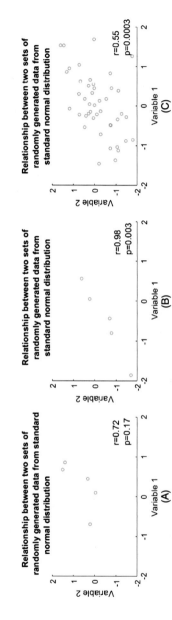

FIGURE 2.12

Random data to show the effect on p-values of higher correlation and use of more data. (A) A scatter plot of five points sampled from a standard normal distribution where the x and y values correlate, but with a random error ($r = 0.72$, $p = 0.17$). (B) The p-value decreases as r increases ($r = 0.98$, $p = 0.003$). (C) The p-value decreases as the number of points increases ($r = 0.55$, $p = 0.0003$).

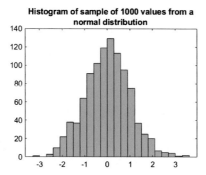

FIGURE 2.13
Example histogram of a sample from a normal distribution.

Fig. 2.12A, there are only five data points and the p-value of 0.17 reveals that there is an almost one in five chance that the 0.72 correlation value occurred just due to random variation in the data and that there was in fact no underlying linear relationship between the two variables. Fig. 2.12B shows the effect of adding a smaller random offset to generate the second variable. The effect is to increase the correlation and decrease the p-value ($r = 0.98$, $p = 0.003$). This illustrates that the p-value is a function of how well the data fit to a straight line. Fig. 2.12C shows what happens when we use the same level of random offset as Fig. 2.12A but add more data points (fifty instead of five). The r value of 0.55 is slightly weaker than that in the left plot but the p-value of 0.0003 is now much lower. This shows that the p-value is also a function of how many data points are involved.

We will cover p-values in more detail in Chapter 5 when we discuss hypothesis testing.

2.4.2 Spearman's Rank Correlation Coefficient

Pearson's correlation coefficient, detailed in the previous section, should only be used if our data values are discrete or continuous and are *normally distributed*. We will cover what being normally distributed means and how to test whether data are normally distributed much more thoroughly from Chapter 4 onwards. However, as a brief introduction, Fig. 2.13 shows a histogram of data that are normally distributed. The histogram is symmetric, follows a bell-shaped curve, and has few outliers.

If the data are ranked or are not normally distributed, then Spearman's rank correlation coefficient[2] should be used to calculate a measure of correlation. The choice between Pearson's and Spearman's correlation coefficients can be

---

[2]This was devised by and named after Charles Spearman; see the *Famous Statistician* at the end of this chapter.

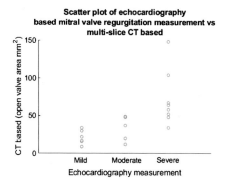

FIGURE 2.14

Scatter plot of mitral valve regurgitation severity: echocardiography measurements (x-axis) and new multislice CT measurements (y-axis).

thought of as being approximately equivalent to choosing between the median/IQR and the mean/standard deviation as explained in Chapter 1. In the same manner as the median and IQR, Spearman's rank correlation coefficient works on the *ranked* values of the data (i.e. not the actual data values themselves, but how they are ranked within the data set in order of value). Therefore, given two sets of discrete/continuous paired variables x_i and $y_i, i = 1, \ldots, n$ (n is the sample size), these are first converted into ranked positions R_i and S_i. Spearman's rank correlation coefficient r_s can then be calculated as follows:

$$r_s = 1 - \frac{6 \sum_{i=1}^{n} D_i^2}{n^3 - n}, \quad \text{where} \quad D_i = R_i - S_i. \tag{2.5}$$

To illustrate, let us consider an example. Mitral regurgitation (backward flow through the mitral valve of the heart) is routinely detected using Doppler echocardiography. However, it can be difficult to quantify the severity of the regurgitation using echocardiography. Researchers have proposed a new method to quantify regurgitation using newly developed multislice computed tomography (CT) scanners. The researchers propose to use the high temporal and spatial resolution of multislice CT to measure the area of the mitral valve that remains open when it should be closed due to left ventricle contraction. The researchers believe that their new method could be a more accurate way to quantify the severity of regurgitation. As a first step, they want to check whether values obtained with their new method correlate well with the standard echocardiography measurements. The researchers measure regurgitation severity from 19 patients using both methods, and the results are shown in Fig. 2.14.

Because the echocardiography measurements produced ranked data, Spearman's rank correlation coefficient should be used (as would be the case if either data set was not normally distributed). The result of 0.7894 shows a

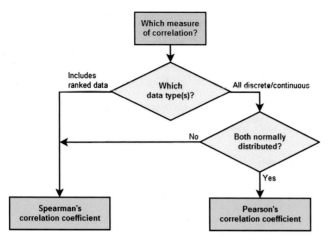

FIGURE 2.15
Summary of choosing an appropriate measure of correlation.

strong correlation, and the low *p*-value of 0.00006 means that the result is very unlikely to have occurred purely by chance. Therefore the researchers can have some confidence that their new measurement method is producing some sensible results.

2.4.3 Which Measure of Correlation to Use?

To summarize, we have introduced two measures of correlation for quantifying the dependency of the value of one variable on that of another. Pearson's correlation coefficient should only be used with discrete or continuous normally distributed variables. If either of the variables is not normally distributed, or if at least one of the variables is ranked, then Spearman's correlation coefficient should be used. The concept of correlation is only meaningful if the data are at least ranked (i.e. not categorical). The flow chart in Fig. 2.15 summarizes some of the factors to consider when choosing a measure of correlation.

2.5 REGRESSION ANALYSIS

Regression analysis deals with methods to fit models to statistical data. Bivariate regression models can be used to predict the value of the first variable (the dependent variable) given the value of the second variable (the independent variable). The performance of the model will depend upon the amount of correlation: if a correlation of $r = 1$ or $r = -1$ is obtained, then the model should be perfect. If the correlation coefficient is zero ($r = 0$), then the model will be useless, that is, have no predictive power.

We shall use the following example to demonstrate linear regression. Table 2.4 shows data gathered by a hospital Accident & Emergency department, who

Table 2.4 Record of number of patients treated by a hospital Accident & Emergency department and maximum daily temperature over ten consecutive days.

Number of patients	294	344	360	417	359	422	333	443	350	401
Max temperature	19	23	20	24	21	26	20	25	22	29

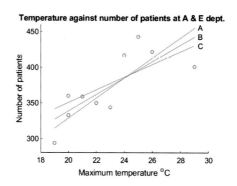

FIGURE 2.16

Scatter plot of number of patients at hospital Accident & Emergency department plotted against maximum daily temperature. Three possible best-fit lines are drawn: A, B and C.

recorded the maximum daily temperature and the number of patients they treated over ten consecutive days.

Fig. 2.16 shows a scatter plot of these data, and three possible linear models: the lines labeled A, B, and C. By eye, each of these lines looks to be a reasonable match to the data. How can we mathematically obtain a *best-fit* line? In what sense does such a line "best fit"?

The most commonly used method is to find a line that minimizes the sum of squared errors between the model and the data values. Starting with a set of pairs of data values x_i and y_i, $i = 1, \ldots, n$ (n = sample size), we can define our linear model by two parameters a and b such that

$$y_i = a + bx_i + \epsilon_i, \qquad (2.6)$$

and the best-fit solution will be defined as the solution of

$$\min \sum_i^n \epsilon_i^2 = \min \sum_i^n (y_i - a - bx_i)^2. \qquad (2.7)$$

This minimum can be found by partial differentiation with respect to a and b and equating to zero. The result after tidying up is:

$$b = \frac{\sum_i^n y_i x_i - n\bar{x}\bar{y}}{\sum_i^n x_i^2 - n\bar{x}^2}, \qquad (2.8)$$

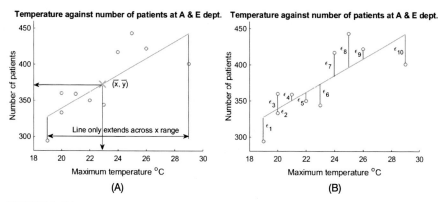

FIGURE 2.17

Regression analysis. (A) The best-fit line goes through the point that represents the mean value of both variables. The extent of the line should be limited by the x range of the data. (B) The values that are minimized ($\min \sum_i^n \epsilon_i^2$). The lines show the values of ϵ_i for each data point, $i = 1, \ldots, 10$.

$$a = \bar{y} - b\bar{x}. \tag{2.9}$$

The differences between the model predictions and the data values, ϵ_i, are often referred to as *residual errors* or just *residuals*. The root mean square value of these residuals is often used as a measure of how well the model fits the data.

The actual best-fit line for this example is shown in Fig. 2.17A, and the parameters of the line are $a = 108.4477$, $b = 11.5219$. Note that the line goes through the point that represents the mean values of both variables, that is, $(\bar{x}, \bar{y})$. This line should not be drawn outside the range of the data on the x-axis. Outside of this range of the x variable we would be using the line to *extrapolate* the relationship *outside of* our known data values. Extrapolation is far more prone to errors than *interpolation*, which means using the model *within* the recorded data values. For example, there may be a temperature above which many more patients will report to the department with heat stroke. This will not be apparent from the data that we currently have, and so our model will not be able to predict it. Note also that the regression process minimizes the squares of the vertical distances between the data points and the best-fit line, as shown in Fig. 2.17B.

2.5.1 Using the Best-Fit Line to Make Predictions

Making predictions with the best-fit line is simply a matter of inserting the known value for one variable into Eq. (2.6) and then calculating the corresponding value of the other variable. For example, if the weather forecast indicated that the temperature was going to be 28 °C, the predicted number of

Table 2.5 Results of an experiment to determine how radioactive activity decreases with respect to time.

Time (mins)	0	10	20	30	40	50	60
Activity (10^3 Bq)	9878	4809	2567	1150	720	405	226

patients would be calculated as:

$$\begin{aligned} \text{patients} &= 108.4477 + 11.5219 \times \text{temperature} \\ &= 108.4477 + 11.5219 \times 28 = 431. \end{aligned}$$

2.5.2 Fitting Nonlinear Models

Sometimes (particularly in experimental studies) a particular relationship between the two variables is expected. We may know this relationship from theory or from past research. If the expected relationship is nonlinear, then a best-fit line can be calculated by using the expected relationship to transform our data so that they should be linearly related and then fitting a straight line to the data as described in the previous section.

For example, Table 2.5 shows radioactivity counts measured by a researcher at 10 minute intervals. From the theory of radioactive decay the researcher knows that the activity A should follow an exponential decay curve, and so

$$A = A_0 e^{-\lambda t}, \tag{2.10}$$

where A_0 is the activity at time $t = 0$, and λ is the decay constant. The researcher would like to calculate the value of λ by fitting a best-fit line to the data. The result of taking logarithms of both sides of Eq. (2.10) is

$$\log(A) = \log(A_0) - \lambda t, \tag{2.11}$$

which shows that there should be a linear relationship between $\log(A)$ and t and that λ will equal the negative slope of the best-fit line.

Following the same approach as before, we find that the decay constant $\lambda = 0.0627$, and $\log(A_0) = 9.1061$. Therefore, the exponential-decay-model best-fit line is

$$A = 9010 \times e^{-0.0627t}. \tag{2.12}$$

This model line is plotted in Fig. 2.18, where it can be seen to agree well with the experimental data.

2.5.3 Fitting Higher-Order Polynomials

The examples above all used straight lines as the best-fit model, that is, first-order polynomials. Increasing the order of the polynomial will always result

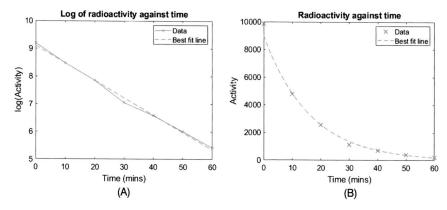

FIGURE 2.18

Fitting nonlinear best-fit models. (A) The solid line shows a plot of the log of the experimental radioactive decay data vs. time. The dashed line is the best-fit line to the data. The line slope equals the negative of the radioactive decay constant. (B) The exponential decay model best-fit line and the original data points.

in a lower residual error because the fitted function has more degrees of freedom. At first glance this appears to be a good thing: the higher-order model will generally have better agreement with our data. However, as the order of the model increases, it becomes more likely that it is fitting to the *errors* in the data rather than the underlying *relationship*. This situation is termed *overfitting* and should be avoided. Fig. 2.19 shows how our model line changes as the polynomial order increases from 1 to 5. The higher-order polynomials fit to the data more accurately, but can we justify producing such a complicated model from just ten data points? The question to ask is "if I was to obtain a new set of data, would I expect to calculate a similar best-fit line?" The answer is probably "yes" for our simple linear model, and probably "no" to definitely "no" for the higher-order models.

From a purely statistical viewpoint, it is good to follow the principle of *Occam's razor* when deciding which order of polynomial to use. Occam's razor essentially asserts that the simplest solution tends to be the right one. Therefore it is good practice to begin with the polynomial order as low as possible and only increase the order when we are convinced that the produced model will have a greater predictive power (i.e. it is not just fitting to errors in the data). Of course, if there is additional knowledge available concerning the relationship between the variables, such as in the previous example where there was a known physical theory about radioactive decay over time, then it is fully justifiable to use this knowledge to form the model.

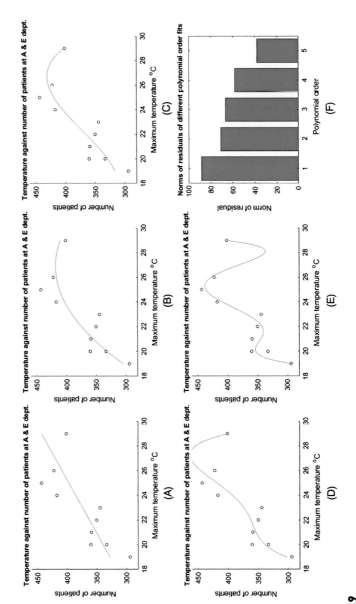

FIGURE 2.19

Overfitting of higher-order polynomials. (A)–(E) Best-fit lines to the same data using polynomials of order 1 to 5. (F) The norm of the res dual values decreases as the polynomial order increases. This is a result of overfitting to errors, not an indication of an improved model.

■ **Activity 2.3**

A student alters the temperature T of a gas 5 times over a range between 275   O2.E
degrees Kelvin (K) to 350 K. At each temperature they measure the pressure
P. The data are shown in the plot below.

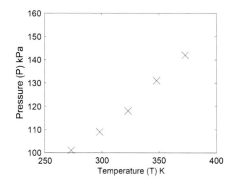

The student uses regression analysis to fit two models to the data:

■ A linear model: $P = 0.416 \times T - 14.168$.
■ A quadratic model: $P = 0.0011 \times T^2 - 0.322 \times T + 103.637$.

The quadratic model has lower residual errors.

1. Use the linear model to predict the pressure at 320 K.
2. Use the linear model to predict the pressure at 400 K.
3. Which of these predictions is likely to be more accurate and why?
4. Is the linear model or the quadratic model more likely to represent the
    underlying relationship between temperature and pressure?
5. Explain why the quadratic model has a lower residual error.
                                                                    ■

2.6 BLAND–ALTMAN ANALYSIS

It is quite common for biomedical engineers to need to be able to compare
the agreement between two methods that claim to make the same measurement. We have seen before how correlation can be used as a way to quantify
this agreement. For example, measurements made by two methods referred to
as Method A and Method B are represented in Fig. 2.20, which shows a scatter
plot of the paired data with the best-fit straight line overlaid on the graph. The
correlation value of $r = 0.9974$ and $p < 0.005$ suggests a strong linear relationship between the data measured using the two methods.

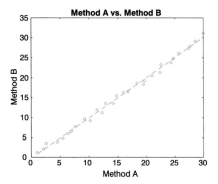

FIGURE 2.20
Scatter plot of paired measurements obtained using both Methods A and B. The dashed line is the best-fit linear regression. The correlation between the methods is $r = 0.9974$ with $p < 0.005$.

2.6.1 The Bland–Altman Plot

While correlation does provide an indicator of agreement, it is based on a study of the relationship between them rather than their comparability. In 1983, Bland and Altman [2] proposed a quantitative measure of agreement that is based on the concept of *limits of agreement*. These limits are based on the mean and standard deviation of the differences between the two measurement approaches. Once again we use a scatter plot, except that in this case the x-axis shows the mean of each pair of measurements, whereas the y-axis represents the difference between them. For the data presented in Fig. 2.20, the corresponding Bland–Altman plot is shown in Fig. 2.21. The distance of the central solid horizontal line from zero represents any *bias* between the two techniques. The upper and lower solid horizontal lines show the 95% *confidence interval of the mean* of the difference between the techniques. The concept of confidence intervals belongs to parametric statistical analysis and is covered in detail in Chapter 4. Simply stated though, the confidence interval (the distance between the upper and lower solid lines) in Fig. 2.21 represents the region within which 95% of the differences lie.

As is often the case in practical statistics, our interpretation of this graph actually depends upon what we know about the problem we are trying to solve. Bland–Altman analysis must be used together with knowledge of the underlying requirements of the situation. These requirements should be based on an understanding of the application and the underlying basic science.

As an example, imaging scientists are developing a new, cheaper and quicker, method for measuring the diameter of tumors in cancer patients. They perform a comparison study of the new technique and their existing approach on a cohort of 40 patients. Current clinical practice requires the technique that they use to be able to measure tumor size to within ± 2 mm. The Bland–Altman

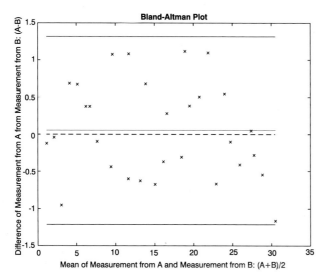

FIGURE 2.21
Bland–Altman plot for the data shown in Fig. 2.20.

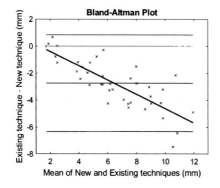

FIGURE 2.22
Bland–Altman plot for the tumor diameter measurement techniques. The red line represents zero difference between the two techniques. The solid black lines are the mean difference and the 95% confidence interval. The bold black line represents the bias, which is dependent on the value.

plot of the results is presented in Fig. 2.22. There are several issues with the new technique that are visualized using this plot.

The key revelation is that the 95% confidence interval of the mean of the difference between the techniques is greater than the 2 mm requirement for clinical practice, suggesting that this technique is not an improvement on the original method. Additionally, the mean difference between the techniques shows a −2.75 mm negative bias of the new technique compared to the existing one, and on closer inspection a trend can be seen (the thicker line in Fig. 2.22). This trend suggests a bias in the new technique that is dependent on the value. Of course, this bias could be calibrated given sufficient data and available calibration tools. Interestingly, the correlation value of $r = 0.9131$ and $p < 0.005$ still suggests a strong linear relationship between the two methods.

■ **Activity 2.4**

O2.F   Look again at the data presented in Fig. 2.22. Do you think that once the new method has been calibrated (i.e. the bias removed), it would be acceptable in clinical practice?   ■

2.7 SUMMARY

There are a number of different ways to display bivariate data. Several common methods have been described in this chapter. It is important to be aware of the range of possible methods, so that the most appropriate method can be selected. Using graphical techniques to visualize data provides powerful ways to reveal and investigate any trends in the data, and to help discover any errors that could have occurred during data acquisition.

Covariance is a numerical measure that can be used to quantify how strongly the variations of pairs of variables are related. A covariance matrix contains the covariances between all pairs of variables in multivariate data sets.

Correlation is another measure of how closely linked two variables are. It is important to remember that the significance of a correlation also depends on the number of data values involved in the calculation. This is expressed by the p-value. Also, it is a very common mistake to believe that correlation implies a "causal link" between the two variables, that is, changing the value of one variable will cause the other to change. Correlation does not mean causation, as correlation can also result from the presence of a third confounding variable, or just simply by chance.

Two measures of correlation have been introduced in this chapter. Pearson's correlation coefficient should be used with discrete or continuous normally distributed data. If either data set is not normally distributed or contains ranked data, then Spearman's rank correlation coefficient should be used.

Although correlation does not show that altering one variable can allow control of the other, a strong correlation does imply that knowledge of one variable can allow prediction of the second variable. This prediction can be achieved by fitting a model to the data. This process is known as regression. Regression typically minimizes the mean squared error between the chosen model and the data values. Simple linear models are the most commonly used. More complex models should only be used if they greatly improve predictive power, or if the model is based on a known mathematical relationship between the variables.

When comparing two measurement techniques, we can use correlation to provide an indication of their agreement. However, a Bland–Altman plot can provide further insight into any potential disagreement by providing a visual representation of differences between the two approaches. It should be noted, though, that only with additional prior knowledge can such a plot be used to determine whether this agreement is acceptable or otherwise.

2.8 DESCRIPTIVE BIVARIATE AND MULTIVARIATE STATISTICS USING MATLAB

2.8.1 Visualizing Bivariate Data

Joint Contingency Tables:

The MATLAB `crosstab` command can be used to compute the values for a joint contingency table. There is no built-in function for displaying these values in a figure window. The `frequencyTable` function that we have provided below was used to generate the joint contingency table shown in Fig. 2.1. This code is available through the book's web site.

```
function [] = frequencyTable(x, y)
% usage:
% [] = frequencyTable( x, y )
% x,y input variables: must have the same length
% output is frequency table of unique values within x and y
table = crosstab(x, y)
xlabels = unique(x, 'stable');
ylabels = unique(y, 'stable');
f = figure('Position',[200 200 400 150]);
t = uitable('Parent',f,'Data',table, ...
    'ColumnName',ylabels,'Rowname', xlabels, ...
    'Position',[20 20 360 100]);
end
```

Scatter Plots:

```
scatter(x, y)
```

Produces a scatter plot from the (equal length) vectors x and y. For example, the code listed below was used to generate Fig. 2.2.

```
load('fortyStudentDistanceData.mat')
load('fortyStudentHeightData.mat')
scatter(heights, distance);
ylabel('Distance travelled to University (km)')
xlabel('Height (cm)');
title('Scatter plot of height vs. distance traveled');
```

2D Histograms:

```
n = hist3(x)
```

Creates a bivariate histogram plot of x(:,1) and x(:,2). The optional return argument n is a 2D array containing the counts in each bin. As illustrated in the code below, which was used to generate Figs. 2.3 and 2.4, this can be used to produce an intensity plot using imagesc.

```
load('fortyStudentDistanceData.mat')
load('fortyStudentHeightData.mat')
heightNdistance=[heights, distance];
%for intensity plot
histArray = hist3(heightNdistance);
colormap(gray);
imagesc(histArray);
%for 3D plot
figure;
hist3(heightNdistance)
xlabel('Height (cm)');
ylabel('Distance traveled to University (km)');
title('2D histogram of height vs distance traveled');
```

Line graphs:

The line graph shown in Fig. 2.5 was produced using the MATLAB plot command as illustrated below.

```
inr = [2.4 2.8 2.3 2.7 2.6 3.0 3.1 2.9 3.2 3.3 3.7 4.1];
day = [1 8 15 22 29 36 43 50 57 64 71 78]
plot(day, inr, '-k');
title('INR value against time');
xlabel('Time (days)');
ylabel('INR');
```

2.8.2   Covariance

The covariance between two variables, or the covariance matrix of vectors of multivariate data, can be computed using the MATLAB cov function. The code listing shown below illustrates both cases.

```
% define two (random) variables, each with 10 values
x = randn(10,1);
y = randn(10,1);

% compute covariance between them
c = cov(x, y)
% the result is a symmetric 2x2 matrix, in which the
% leading diagonal contains the variance of
% the two variables, and the off-diagonal values
% represent the covariance between them.
```

```
% define vector of 4 variables, 10 samples
x = randn(10,4);
cm = cov(x)
% the result is a 4x4 covariance matrix
```

2.8.3   Correlation

```
[r, p] = corr(x, y, 'type', t)
```

Computes Pearson's or Spearman's correlation coefficient between the equal length vectors x and y. The return arguments r and p are the correlation and the *p*-value respectively. If the optional extra argument pair 'type', t is omitted, then the function computes Pearson's correlation coefficient. If the arguments are included and the value 'Spearman' used in place of t, then Spearman's correlation coefficient is computed.

The following examples illustrate the calculation of both Pearson's and Spearman's correlation coefficients.

Pearson's Correlation Coefficient:

The following code computes the Pearson's correlation between the weekly alcohol and tobacco expenditure data presented in Section 2.4.1. The datasets "Region.mat", "weeklyAlcoholSpend.mat" and "weeklyTobaccoSpend.mat" contain these data and are available from the book's web site.

```
%load data
load('weeklyAlcoholSpend.mat');
load('weeklyTobaccoSpend.mat');
load('Region.mat');

% Pearson's correlation including the outlier
[r, p] = corr(weeklyAlcoholSpend, weeklyTobaccoSpend)
% r = 0.2236, p = 0.5087

% use the fact that the potential outlier is the only
% point with alcohol expenditure less than 4.2 to
% find its array index
outlierIndex = find(weeklyAlcoholSpend<4.2);
Region(outlierIndex) % ans = 'NorthernIreland'

% see what value of Pearson's correlation coefficient we
% obtain without the data from NorthernIreland
dataWithoutNI =  find(weeklyAlcoholSpend>4.2);
[r, p] = corr(weeklyAlcoholSpend(dataWithoutNI), ...
              weeklyTobaccoSpend(dataWithoutNI))
% r = 0.7843, p = 0.0072
```

Spearman's Correlation Coefficient:

The following code computes the Spearman's correlation coefficient between the Doppler echocardiography and multislice CT based estimates of mitral valve area, as presented in Section 2.4.2. The data files "DopplerGrading.mat" and "CTvalveArea.mat" are available from the book's web site.

```
%load data
load('DopplerGrading.mat')
load('CTvalveArea.mat')
%calculate correlation
[r,p] = corr(DopplerGrading, CTvalveArea, 'type', 'Spearman')
%r = 0.7894, p = 5.8605e-05
```

2.8.4   Calculating Best-Fit Lines

```
[p, S] = polyfit(x, y, o)
```

Computes the best-fit line of order o between the data in the arrays x and y. The first return argument p contains the polynomial coefficients: $p(1) = b$ is the slope, and $p(2) = a$ is the intercept of the line (see Eq. (2.6)). The second (optional) return argument S is a MATLAB *structure* that contains multiple named data fields. One of these is the field normr, which is the norm of the residual values, that is, $normr = \sqrt{\sum_{i=1}^{n} \epsilon_i^2}$.

For example, the following code fits a straight line between the patient and temperature data presented in Section 2.5 and then plots the original data and the best-fit line. Note the use of the polyval function that evaluates a polynomial at given value(s).

```
patients = [294 344 360 417 359 422 333 443 350 401];
temperature = [19 23 20 24 21 26 20 25 22 29];
[p, S] = polyfit(temperature, patients, 1)

scatter(temperature, patients);
% find x and y points on line at max and min range of x data
xline = [min(temperature), max(temperature)];
yline = polyval(p, xline);

% plot best fit line
hold on
line(xline, yline)
```

The same commands can be used to fit nonlinear models. The following MAT-LAB code was used to produce the plots shown in Fig. 2.18 to calculate the best-fit line and so find λ.

```
% load in the data sets
load('time.mat');
load('activity.mat');

% plot log(Activity) vs time
plot(time, log(activity), 'x-');
```

```
% calculate best fit line parameters
p = polyfit(time, log(activity), 1);
%p = -0.0627    9.1061
xline = [min(time), max(time)];
yline = [polyval(p,min(time)), polyval(p,max(time))];

% plot best fit line
hold on
plot(xline, yline, '--')
xlabel('Time (mins)');
ylabel('log(Activity)');
title('Log of radioactivity against time');
legend('Data', 'Best fit line');

% plot exponential relationship
figure
plot(time, activity, 'x');
hold on;
mintime=min(time); maxtime=max(time);
times=mintime:0.1:maxtime;
plot(times, exp(polyval(p, times)), '--')
xlabel('Time (mins)');
ylabel('Activity');
title('Radioactivity against time');
legend('Data', 'Best fit line');
```

2.8.5 Bland–Altman Analysis

There is no built-in function for producing a Bland–Altman plot in MATLAB. The following code, which is available from the book's web site, illustrates how to produce one and was used to generate Fig. 2.22.

```
% load data
load('BlandAltman002.mat')

% compute means and differences
means = mean([A;B]);
diffs = A-B;
% 95% confidence limits
meanDiff = mean(diffs);
stdDiff = std(diffs);
CR = [meanDiff + 1.96 * stdDiff, meanDiff - 1.96 * stdDiff];
% work out the linear fit coefficients
pMD = polyfit(means,diffs,1);

% Bland–Altman plot
figure(2)
plot(means,diffs,'kx')
hold on
% plot confidence limits
plot(means, ones(1,length(means)).*CR(1),'k-');
plot(means, ones(1,length(means)).*CR(2),'k-');
```

```
plot(means,zeros(1,length(means)),'r-.');
% plot trend
xline = [min(means), max(means)];
yline = [polyval(pMD,min(means)), polyval(pMD,max(means))];
plot(xline, yline, 'k','LineWidth',2)
% plot meanDiff
plot(means,ones(1,length(means))*meanDiff,'k');
xlim([1 13]);
xlabel('Mean of New and Existing techniques (mm)');
ylabel('Existing technique - New technique (mm)');
title('Bland-Altman Plot')
```

2.9 FURTHER RESOURCES

- Good basic tutorials on Pearson's correlation coefficient and Spearman's rank correlation coefficient can be found here:
  https://statistics.laerd.com/statistical-guides/spearmans-rank-order-correlation-statistical-guide.php,
  https://statistics.laerd.com/statistical-guides/pearson-correlation-coefficient-statistical-guide.php
- "Understanding Bland–Altman Analysis", a paper by Davide Giavarina [3] is a nice explanation of the use and interpretation of Bland–Altman plots.

2.10 EXERCISES

Perform the following tasks using MATLAB.

- **Exercise 2.1**

O2.A, O2.B, O2.C

The enlargement of brain ventricles has been proposed as an indicator of Alzheimer's disease progression. Biomedical engineers have produced software systems which allow the change in size of brain ventricles to be accurately measured from 3D magnetic resonance (MR) scans. The file "AlzheimersData.mat" contains the result of a study in which 18 Alzheimer's patients had their disease progression measured using two methods, a "task-based" method and ventricle size. Each patient was measured at two time points, and the file "AlzheimersData.mat" shows the change in the "task-based" method (first column, positive values show symptoms becoming worse) and the change in ventricle size (second column, in cm^3). Investigate how strongly these measures are correlated as follows:

1. Visualize the data using a scatter plot. What does the scatter plot show?
2. Calculate the Pearson's correlation coefficient between the values of the two methods. What does this mean?
3. Calculate the associated p-value. What does this mean?

4. Calculate the covariance matrix of the values of the two methods. What does this mean?
5. From the scatter plot, one data point looks like it has a major impact on the correlation value. Try removing this point and recalculating the correlation coefficient and p-value.

■

■ Exercise 2.2

Using the same Alzheimer's data set "AlzheimersData.mat" described in the previous exercise:

O2.D

1. Calculate the equation of the best-fit line through the data.
2. If an Alzheimer's patient increased their task-based score by one, then how much would you predict their brain ventricle size would increase by (in cm^3)?
3. Visualize the data using a scatter plot. (Although this has already been done in Exercise 2.1, always visualizing your data is a good habit to get into.)
4. Use xlim and ylim to increase the range of the scatter plot so that all of the data are clearly visible in the plot.
5. Plot the best-fit line on the scatter plot.
6. Predict the most likely change in ventricle size that would occur if a patient's task-based score increased by 10.
7. Use the *Basic fitting window* (found under *Tools*, which is located on the top menu bar on MATLAB figures) to fit higher-order polynomials to the data. Click on the → button and observe how the "Norm of residuals" decreases as the polynomial degree increases. Which degree of polynomial should be used to represent the relationship between the variables?

■

■ Exercise 2.3

A study is investigating the link between alcohol use and hypertension (high blood pressure). Data have been gathered from 50 volunteers. The data consist of the number of units of alcohol consumed per day, and the end systolic blood pressure (in mmHg). These data are contained in the files "alcohol.mat" and "blood_pressure.mat".

O2.A, O2.C, O2.D, O2.E

1. Write code to visualize the relationship between alcohol units and blood pressure using a suitable method.
2. Compute the correlation coefficient between daily alcohol units and blood pressure. Also determine the probability that this correlation

value might have occurred by chance. Comment on the results. (You can assume that both sets of data are normally distributed.)

3. Use linear regression to calculate the best-fit straight line between alcohol units and blood pressure. Plot this line on the same visualization that you produced in the first part of this exercise.

4. Based on your answer to the previous part, answer the following questions about these data:

   a. Can you conclude that consuming more alcohol causes an increase in blood pressure?

   b. What would be the estimated blood pressure for an individual who consumed 5 units of alcohol per day?

   c. An individual has an end systolic blood pressure of 120 mmHg. How many alcohol units would you estimate that they consume per day? Round your answer to the nearest integer.

■ **Exercise 2.4**

O2.A, O2.C, O2.D, O2.E

A research team is evaluating a new vaccine for malaria. The vaccine works by injecting cytotoxic lymphocyte cells that attack infected liver cells. The team has tested the vaccine on a cohort of 1000 subjects considered to be at high risk of infection from malaria. The vaccine was administered to half of the subjects (randomly selected), and a placebo was administered to the other half. Six months later data were gathered about whether each of the subjects had contracted malaria or not.

These data are available to you in the file "malaria_data.mat". The file contains two variables:

■ `vaccine`: Was the subject given the vaccine or a placebo? ("V" = vaccine, "P" = placebo)

■ `malaria`: Did the subject contract malaria? ("N" = no, "Y" = yes)

Based on these data, perform the following task.

1. Write code to load the data into the MATLAB workspace and produce an appropriate single visualization that summarizes the data in both the `vaccine` and `malaria` variables.

The research team is also interested in analyzing potential side effects of the new vaccine, in particular its possible effect on liver function. Liver function can be quantified using a blood test to determine the level of alanine transaminase (ALT), which is an enzyme found in liver cells. When liver function drops, the level of ALT typically rises.

To assess potential side effects of the vaccine, the team have gathered data of lymphocyte level and ALT level from the 500 subjects who were given the vaccine. These data are contained in the variables `lymphocyte` and `ALT` in the file "vaccine_side_effects.mat". The lymphocyte levels represent the number of cells per cubic millimeter, and the ALT levels are in international units/liter (IU/L).

Based on these data, perform the following tasks.

2. Produce *two different* visualizations that each show the relationship between the `lymphocyte` and `ALT` variables.
3. Compute a best-fit straight line between the lymphocyte level and the ALT level data. (You do not need to visualize the line, just compute its polynomial coefficients.)
4. Answer the following questions. Use the correct units in your answers and state any concerns that you might have about any of the answers.
   a. What ALT level would you expect for an individual who has 3500 lymphocyte cells per cubic millimeter?
   b. What ALT level would you expect for an individual who has 6000 lymphocyte cells per cubic millimeter?
   c. What lymphocyte level would you expect for an individual who has an ALT level of 20 IU/L?

   ■

■ **Exercise 2.5**

Load in the data from the file "CancerImaging.mat". These data were used to generate the Bland–Altman plot shown in Fig. 2.22 and contain paired data on tumor sizes (in mm) for a cohort of 40 patients.

O2.A, O2.C, O2.D, O2.F, O2.G

1. Visualize these data using a scatter plot.
2. Calculate a correlation coefficient between the two techniques.
3. Generate a Bland–Altman plot of the data. This should be similar to Fig. 2.22, and you can base your code on that provided in Section 2.8.5.
4. Calculate the equation of the best-fit line to the difference data.
5. Use the equation of the best-fit line to correct for the bias in the new measurement technique.
6. Generate a new Bland–Altman plot comparing the "calibrated" new technique against the original technique.
7. Comment on whether the agreement between the techniques is acceptable based upon the clinical requirement that tumor size should be measured to within ±2 mm.

   ■

FAMOUS STATISTICIAN: CHARLES SPEARMAN

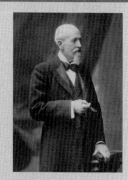

Charles Spearman is quite unusual in the history of statistics because he never really considered himself to be a statistician at all. However, the achievements for which he is perhaps best remembered today lie in the field of statistics. Spearman was born in 1863 in London. He did not show any early desire for an academic career and served 15 years in the British army. However, in 1897 he resigned from the army and started studying for a PhD in experimental psychology.

Because he had no conventional qualifications he was unable to do so in the UK, so moved to Leipzig in Germany where the entrance requirements were, at the time, less stringent. After being briefly called back to the army to serve in the South African war, he completed his PhD in 1906. He subsequently worked in a psychological laboratory at University College London. Up until this point his life and work had been interesting but unremarkable. However, in 1904 (whilst still studying for his PhD) he published two remarkable papers that caught the attention of the most famous statisticians in the world. The papers dealt mainly with ways of measuring the similarity between different sets of data. Contained within these papers was a description of what is now known as Spearman's rank correlation coefficient, which has proved very influential and is still in common use today. However, also contained within these papers was a direct criticism of the work of Karl Pearson (see Chapter 1's *Famous Statistician*). This criticism drew a blistering response from Pearson and resulted in a bitter and lifelong feud between the two men. Although Spearman achieved most recognition in his day for his statistical work, he regarded this work as subordinate to his quest for the fundamental laws of psychology. He died aged 82 in London in 1945.

CHAPTER 3

Descriptive Statistics III: ROC Analysis

LEARNING OBJECTIVES

At the end of this chapter you should be able to:

O3.A *Calculate sensitivity and specificity values by hand and using MATLAB, and explain what they mean*

O3.B *Calculate positive and negative predictive values by hand and using MATLAB, and explain what they mean*

O3.C *Explain the utility of an ROC curve and produce one using MATLAB or sketch one by hand*

O3.D *Use the Youden index to select the best test, both by hand and using MATLAB*

3.1 INTRODUCTION

This chapter introduces the notation used to evaluate devices or new tests. Very few devices or tests work 100% of the time. We describe methods that can be used to characterize the performance of a device or test, and explore how to manipulate the parameters of a test to obtain best performance.

Terms such as *false positives, false negatives, true positives* and *true negatives* will be introduced. We will learn how these new terms can be combined to calculate *sensitivity* and *specificity* and from these construct a *receiver operating characteristic* (ROC) curve.

Some of the above terms may be familiar or even seem fairly self-explanatory. However, without precise understanding of their meaning, confusion can occur. For example, consider a test to detect a disease that has a false positive rate[1] of 5%. If previous studies have shown that the prevalence of the disease in the population is 1/1000, then what is the probability that a randomly selected individual who tests positive actually has the disease?

---

[1]The *false positive rate* is the percentage of people who test positive but do not actually have the disease.

Statistics for Biomedical Engineers and Scientists. https://doi.org/10.1016/B978-0-08-102939-8.00012-8

Table 3.1 Presentation of *true positives* (TP), *false positives* (FP), *true negatives* (TN) and *false negatives* (FN) as a joint contingency table. GT stands for ground truth.

	GT positive	**GT negative**	**Total**
Test positive	TP	FP	TP + FP
Test negative	FN	TN	FN + TN
Total	TP + FN	FP + TN	TP + FP + FN + TN

This question was originally posed to students and staff at a top medical school in 1978 by Casscells et al. [4], and only 18% of the participants answered correctly.

The correct answer is that approximately 2% of the time will an individual who tests positive actually have the disease.

■ **Activity 3.1**

O3.A, O3.B   If you are confident, then have a go at solving Casscells' problem for yourself. If not, read through Section 3.2 first and then have a go.

To reiterate the problem: A test for a disease has a false positive rate of 5%. It is known that the disease has a prevalence in the population of 1/1000. An individual receives a positive test result. What is the probability that they actually have the disease?   ■

3.2   NOTATION

Given results from investigating a new test or device and a set of *ground truth* (GT) results,[2] we can calculate the following quantities:

- *True positives* (TP): The number of times the new test and the ground truth both returned a positive result.
- *False positives* (FP): The number of times the new test returned a positive result but the ground truth returned a negative result.
- *False negatives* (FN): The number of times the new test returned a negative result but the ground truth returned a positive result.
- *True negatives* (TN): The number of times the new test and the ground truth both returned a negative result.

These values are often summarized as shown in Table 3.1, similar to the joint contingency tables that we introduced in Section 2.2.1.

---

[2]This refers to perfectly correct results, also often referred to as *gold standard* results.

3.2.1 Sensitivity and Specificity

The above terms (TP, FP, FN and TN) can be used to define two additional terms that are often used to describe the performance of a test:

- *Sensitivity* (Se): $Se = TP/(TP + FN)$
- *Specificity* (Sp): $Sp = TN/(TN + FP)$

Consider the following example to help describe the meaning of these two new terms. Researchers have devised a new test for a disease. They already have a ground truth test, which always produces accurate results, but it is very expensive and has some side effects, so they would like to replace it with a cheaper and safer alternative. The sensitivity of the new test is the percentage chance of it giving a correct result given that an individual has the disease (i.e. according to the ground truth). Therefore, a high sensitivity means that the test is very likely to detect the disease. The specificity of the test is the percentage chance of it being correct given that an individual does *not* have the disease. Therefore a high specificity means that the test is unlikely to indicate that the individual has the disease by mistake (i.e. when in fact they are healthy).

Ideally, a test should have a high sensitivity and specificity ($Se = Sp = 1$). It should be noted, though, that these two terms are interrelated and should always be reported together. It is very easy to produce a trivial test that has perfect sensitivity; we could just say that everyone has the disease (then $FN = TN = 0$ since there are no negative results, and $Se = 1$, however, $Sp = 0$). Similarly, a trivial test can be produced that has perfect specificity, by simply stating that nobody has the disease (then $FP = TP = 0$ as there are no positives, and $Sp = 1$, however, $Se = 0$). It is more challenging to design a test that has both high sensitivity and specificity.

3.2.2 Positive and Negative Predictive Values

The same terms (TP, FP, FN and TN) can also be used to define two more commonly used values:

- *Positive Predictive Value* (PPV): $PPV = TP/(TP + FP)$
- *Negative Predictive Value* (NPV): $NPV = TN/(TN + FN)$

Continuing with the same example as before, the positive predictive value is the percentage chance of the test being correct, given that it returned a positive result. It shows the power of the test to give positive predictions. Therefore, if our new test had a high PPV and our individual tested positive for the disease, then the individual would be very likely to have the disease. The negative predictive value is the percentage chance of the test being correct, given that it returned a negative result. It shows the power of the test to give negative pre-

Table 3.2 Summary of the results of using ultrasound color Doppler imaging for differential diagnosis of lesions in the thyroid. The ground truth (GT) is obtained by taking a biopsy.

	GT positive	GT negative	Total
Test positive (Area $\geq 4\,\text{mm}^2$)	20	8	28
Test negative (Area $< 4\,\text{mm}^2$)	10	24	34
Total	30	32	62

dictions. Therefore, if our new test had a high NPV and our individual tested negative for the disease, then they would be very unlikely to have the disease.

3.2.3 Example Calculation of Se, Sp, PPV and NPV

A new ultrasound imaging test is proposed with the aim of differentiating benign from malignant lesions in the thyroid. The test involves deriving a surrogate measure for blood volume from the cross-sectional area of color Doppler signals detected within a lesion. The new test is compared against histological results obtained from a biopsy. Using an area of $4\,\text{mm}^2$ as the cutoff threshold in the ultrasound images to differentiate between benign and malignant lesions, there were 20 true positives, 8 false positives, 24 true negatives and 10 false negatives. These results are summarized in Table 3.2.

Substituting the values from Table 3.2 into the equations from the two previous sections results in:

- Se $= 0.67$
- Sp $= 0.75$
- PPV $= 0.71$
- NPV $= 0.71$

These values can be interpreted as follows:

- If an individual who was tested has a malignant lesion, then the ultrasound-based test is 67% likely to detect it (Se $= 0.67$).
- If an individual who was tested does not have a malignant lesion, then the ultrasound test has a 75% chance of correctly identifying the lesion as benign (Sp $= 0.75$). Therefore the ultrasound test has a 25% chance of incorrectly saying a person has a malignant lesion when in fact they are healthy.
- If the ultrasound-based test returns a positive result, then the individual is 71% likely to have a malignant lesion (PPV $= 0.71$).
- If the test returns a negative result, then the individual is 71% likely to have a benign lesion (NPV $= 0.71$).

■ **Activity 3.2**

A patient is informed by their doctor that they have tested positive for prostate cancer.

O3.A, O3.B

In a recently published retrospective study of 10000 subjects who had the same test, 420 subjects tested positive. Of these 420 subjects, 390 were subsequently confirmed to have cancer through follow-up examinations, while the remainder were given the all-clear. Additionally, 6 of the subjects who returned a negative test for prostate cancer were eventually found to have the disease.

1. Summarize the findings of the study in a joint contingency table.
2. How likely is it that the patient who tested positive actually has cancer?
3. Calculate the sensitivity and specificity of the test and provide an interpretation of the results that you obtain.

■

3.3 ROC CURVES

A test that returns a binary decision (i.e. positive or negative) will often make this decision by applying a threshold to a continuously measured value. Using the ultrasound imaging example from Section 3.2.3, the binary decision was that the patient had either a malignant lesion or a benign lesion. This decision was made by measuring the area of flow in the image and then applying a threshold: if the area was $\geq 4\,\mathrm{mm}^2$, then the test returned a positive result (the patient had a malignant lesion), and if it was $< 4\,\mathrm{mm}^2$, then the test returned a negative result (the patient had a benign lesion). But how was this threshold value of $4\,\mathrm{mm}^2$ obtained? Could a different value potentially provide a more useful test? Plotting an ROC curve can help to answer such questions.

An ROC curve plots the sensitivity against one minus the specificity for a range of threshold values. Even before carrying out any experimentation with our new test, we already know two points on such a graph. These are the two trivial tests discussed in Section 3.2.1, that is, one test always returns a positive result ($\mathrm{Se} = 1$ and $\mathrm{Sp} = 0$), and the other always returns a negative result ($\mathrm{Se} = 0$ and $\mathrm{Sp} = 1$). Additional points are then added after experiments with different thresholds. The first experiment (discussed in Section 3.2.3) used a threshold of $4\,\mathrm{mm}^2$ and resulted in $\mathrm{Se} = 0.67$ and $\mathrm{Sp} = 0.75$. When an increased threshold of $6\,\mathrm{mm}^2$ was applied and the experimental data reprocessed the researchers reported an increased sensitivity $\mathrm{Se} = 0.90$ but a lower specificity $\mathrm{Sp} = 0.50$. The resulting ROC curve based on these values is plotted in Fig. 3.1.

The closer the ROC curve gets to the top left corner of the graph, where $\mathrm{Se} = 1$ and $\mathrm{Sp} = 1$, the better the test can be said to be. The area under the ROC curve is

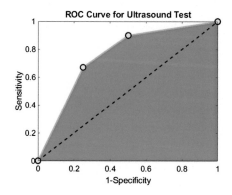

FIGURE 3.1
ROC curve for ultrasound color Doppler test. The dotted line indicates the $x = y$ line. The area under the curve is shaded.

often provided as a measure of how good a test is and can be used to compare two tests.

One method to choose the best threshold value is known as the *Youden index*[3]

$$YI = \max_i(Se_i + Sp_i - 1). \tag{3.1}$$

This term defines the maximum vertical distance of the points on the ROC curve from the $x = y$ line, where the subscript i represents positions along the ROC curve (or in our example each of the different thresholds used). The term $(Se_i + Sp_i - 1)$ will always have a value between 0 and 1, with 1 representing the perfect test.

■ **Activity 3.3**

O3.C, O3.D

Clinical researchers continue with their work on a new ultrasound-image-based test for differential diagnosis of thyroid lesions as presented in Section 3.2.3. They generate the following results using a wider range of thresholds.

Threshold (mm^2)	Sensitivity	Specificity
3	0.4	0.9
4	0.67	0.75
5	0.8	0.65
6	0.9	0.5
7	0.96	0.25

[3]The Youden index is named after its inventor William Youden. See the Famous Statistician at the end of this chapter.

1. Sketch an ROC curve using the results obtained over the range of thresholds.
2. In relation to ROC curves in general, explain the significance of the following:

   - The top left corner.
   - The line of identity, $x = y$.

3. Describe how an ROC curve can be used to find the best threshold for a test. Demonstrate your answer by estimating which of the thresholds tested for the ultrasound imaging example described above is optimum. Explain how the relative cost of false negatives or false positives might change your answer.

3.4 SUMMARY

The sensitivity and specificity, and positive and negative predictive values provide valuable insight into the usefulness of a test. Their correct interpretation is often essential in understanding test results. The sensitivity and specificity of a test used with varying criteria or threshold values can be used to produce an ROC curve that graphically displays the performance of the test and can be useful in determining the best version to use. The Youden index is a quantitative method that can be used to choose the best version. The area under the ROC curve is commonly quoted as a measure of success for a test.

3.5 USING MATLAB FOR ROC ANALYSIS

The calculation of sensitivity, specificity, and positive and negative predictive values do not require any special MATLAB commands.

Also, ROC analysis as described before can be easily performed using standard MATLAB functions. There is built-in functionality in the *Statistics and Machine Learning Toolbox* of MATLAB for ROC analysis, but in this book we rely solely on core MATLAB functionality. The code listing below illustrates the production of an ROC curve using the full data for the ultrasound-based test for lesion malignancy, as presented in Activity 3.3.

```
% define data
Se=[0.4 0.67 0.8 0.9 0.96]
Sp=[0.9 0.75 0.65 0.5 0.25]

% produce ROC curve
figure
h=area(1-[1 Sp 0],[0 Se 1])
h.FaceColor = [0 0.75 0.75];
hold on
```

```
plot([0 1],[0 1],'k—','LineWidth',2)
plot(1—[1 Sp 0],[0 Se 1],'o—',...
    'LineWidth',2,...
    'MarkerSize',10,...
    'MarkerEdgeColor','k',...
    'MarkerFaceColor','y')

% annotations
ylabel('Sensitivity','FontSize',20)
xlabel('1—Specificity','FontSize',20)
title('ROC Curve for ultrasound test');
```

3.6 FURTHER RESOURCES

■ The paper by Zweig and Campbell [5] is a good research paper on the use of ROC analysis.

3.7 EXERCISES

Perform the following tasks using MATLAB.

■ Exercise 3.1

O3.A, O3.B   You have been provided with a function called calcPPVNPV, which takes as inputs values of TP, FP, FN, and TN (see Table 3.1) and returns PPV and NPV values (see Section 3.2.2).

1. Check the function usage using either help or doc.
2. Supply values of TP, FP, FN, and TN from Table 3.2 as the input arguments to calcPPVNPV and check that the results agree with those presented in Section 3.2.3.
3. Write your own function (call it calcSeSp) to calculate sensitivity and specificity that takes values of TP, FP, FN, and TN as input arguments. *(Hint: Instead of starting from scratch, copy "calcPPVNPV.m" to a new file called "calcSeSp.m" and then alter the code in the function.)*
4. Supply values of TP, FP, FN and TN from Table 3.2 as the input arguments to your new function calcSeSp and check that the results agree with those presented in the ultrasound imaging example (see Section 3.2.3).

■

■ Exercise 3.2

O3.C, O3.D   Radiologists are interested in determining whether the time of arrival of an ultrasound imaging contrast agent in the liver of a patient can reveal the presence or otherwise of microscopic metastatic tumors. They have observed that patients with this disease appear to have a much shorter arrival time.

A clinical trial has been performed, and the arrival time of the contrast agent has been recorded in 1000 subjects. The gold standard diagnosis for each patient is obtained through an invasive biopsy.

The data from the trial are stored in the file "ultrasound.mat". The file contains two variables: GroundTruth, which is 1 in the case where the disease was found and 0 otherwise, and TestData, which provides the corresponding time of arrival (in seconds) for each subject.

1. Load the data into the MATLAB workspace and generate an appropriate visualization to enable comparison of the distribution of times for the diseased patients with those of the disease-free subjects. Use this visualization to estimate a threshold in the timing data that might be useful in discriminating between the two subject groups.
2. Using the threshold you estimated in the last part to discriminate between diseased and disease-free subjects, calculate the sensitivity, specificity, positive predictive value and negative predictive value of this new, noninvasive, diagnostic test.
3. Use the full dataset to produce an ROC curve for all possible thresholds.
4. Calculate the optimum threshold assuming that both false positives and false negatives are equally weighted.

∎

◼ Exercise 3.3

In this and the following linked exercises, you will produce a basic *segmentation* tool to extract a femoral implant from a post operative x-ray image (*segmentation* is an image-processing term, which refers to the process of delineating a specific object within an image).

O3.A

Fig. 3.2A shows a postoperative x-ray. Images such as these are used by surgeons to check prosthesis position. Fig. 3.2B shows a ground truth segmentation of the femoral implant. The ground truth was produced using a variety of methods, including some manual drawing. In this case study we will produce an automatic method to segment the implant from the postoperative x-ray. Note that the postoperative x-ray contains a large number of different intensity values, whereas the segmentation image is binary (i.e. only contains the intensities 0 and 1).

As can be seen from Fig. 3.2A, the femoral implant appears as a bright white structure, brighter than most of the image. You will use this information to produce a threshold-based segmentation tool. The provided MATLAB function thresholdImage takes as input an image with a range of intensities and a threshold value. It outputs a binary image that has values of 1 where the input image intensity was above the threshold and 0 where it was less than or equal to the threshold. Fig. 3.2C shows the result of applying the function `thresholdImage` to the postoperative x-ray using a threshold of 180. A reasonable segmentation has been achieved for the lower part of the implant, but the top part is badly segmented. However:

- Would a different threshold have achieved a better job?
- What is the optimal threshold to use?

A skeleton of the main code needed for this case study is provided in the script named "calcROCforImplant.m". Most of the script is commented out. The parts that are not commented out include commands to read an image (`imread`) and to display an image (`imshow`). The `imread` command reads the image into a MATLAB 2D array, so that standard MATLAB commands applicable to matrices or arrays can be used with the image data. The `mat2gray` command scales the intensity range within the image to be from 0 to 1, which is required by `imshow`.

1. Run the script – it should display the three images shown in Fig. 3.2.
2. Try changing the value of the threshold, then rerun the script and see how the intensity-based segmented image changes.
3. Look at the provided, but incomplete, function "calcStats.m". The usage tells you what the function needs to do, and the `for` loops provide an example of how to loop over an image. As shown in the function, values of the input images' intensities can be accessed using the standard MATLAB method for matrices, for example, to access the (i, j)th value of the image matrix you would write `image(i,j)`. Perform the following tasks to complete this function:

   - Use `if` statements to compare the values in the ground truth image (`GTval`) and the segmented image (`testVal`).
   - If both images have the intensity 1, then the true positive variable (`TP`) should be increased by 1.
   - If both images have the intensity 0, then the true negative variable (`TN`) should be increased by 1.
   - If `testVal` equals 0 and `GTval` equals 1, then `FN` should be increased by 1.
   - If `testVal` equals 1 and `GTval` equals 0, then `FP` should be increased by 1.

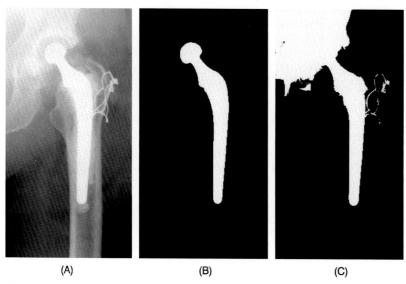

(A)   (B)   (C)

FIGURE 3.2

(A) Postoperative x-ray image after total hip replacement surgery. (B) Ground truth segmentation of hip replacement femoral component. (C) Intensity-based segmentation using a threshold value of 180.

■ Exercise 3.4

Continuing from the previous exercise, you will now generate intensity-based segmentations over a range of different threshold values and calculate the corresponding Se and Sp values.

O3.C

To achieve this, perform the following tasks:

1. Uncomment the lines in the main script "calcROCforImplant.m" that call your new function calcStats (from the previous exercise) and also the function calcSeSp you produced in Exercise 3.1.
2. Run the "calcROCforImplant.m" script with a few different threshold values and observe how the Se and Sp values change. Compare the resulting segmentations with the ground truth segmented image (Fig. 3.2B).
3. Write a loop that goes from the minimum to the maximum intensity value in postOpXray and calculate the values of Se and Sp for every intensity value (i.e. every possible threshold).
4. Run the script with the loop.
5. The values of Se and Sp will be overwritten on each iteration of the loop. You will need these later to plot the ROC curve so store them in a new array variable.

■ **Exercise 3.5**

O3.C, O3.D

Once again we continue the case study from above. In this exercise you will plot the ROC curve and produce a new function to calculate the Youden index (Eq. (3.1)), which will be used to calculate our "best" threshold. To do this, perform the following tasks:

1. Plot the values of Se and Sp that you obtained in the previous exercise as an ROC curve (see Section 3.3).
2. The file "calculateYI.m" contains the first line and usage for a new function. Write this function so that it computes the Youden index (Eq. (3.1)) for each pair of Se and Sp values in the input arrays.
3. Use the new function `calculateYI` to determine the Youden index and Se and Sp values at the optimum threshold (i.e. the maximum Youden index).
4. What is the optimum threshold value?
   (Hint: Just as you saved the values of Se and Sp for each loop iteration, you should store the used threshold values in a separate array to recall the optimum value.)

■

FAMOUS STATISTICIAN: WILLIAM YOUDEN

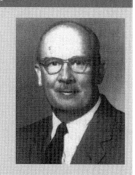

William John Youden was born in 1900 in Australia and lived his early years in Dover in the UK before his family finally moved to the USA. He started to study chemical engineering at the University of Rochester in 1917, before taking a break from his studies to serve in the army in World War I. He graduated with a Batchelor's degree in 1921 and went on to complete a Master's degree and a PhD, both in chemistry. He apparently showed little interest in statistics until he read the book "Statistical Methods" by Ronald Fisher (see Chapter 8's Famous Statistician) in 1928.

He subsequently went on to have a distinguished career in statistics, making major contributions to experimental design and developing what is now known as the Youden index. During World War II, Youden worked for the military as an operations analyst. He spent some time in Britain undertaking war work, mainly investigating the factors that control the accuracy of bombing. In 1974, three years after his death, Youden's final book "Risk, choice and prediction" was published. This book was intended for school children, and Youden wrote in the introduction that it was aimed at anyone "who wants to learn in a relatively painless way how the concept and techniques of statistics can help us better understand today's complex world." He died in 1971 aged 70 in Washington, USA.

CHAPTER 4

Inferential Statistics I: Basic Concepts

LEARNING OBJECTIVES

At the end of this chapter, you should be able to:

O4.A *Explain the role of inferential statistics within the wider field of statistics*

O4.B *Describe the meaning of probability and apply the multiplication and addition rules to determine probabilities of multiple events*

O4.C *Describe the relationship between the probability distribution of a population and the probability distribution of mean values of samples from the population*

O4.D *Describe the meaning of the standard error of the mean and compute it by hand and using MATLAB*

O4.E *Describe the meaning of confidence intervals and compute them by hand and using MATLAB*

4.1 INTRODUCTION

The first three chapters of this book have covered *descriptive statistics*, which enable us to summarize and describe our sample data. In the next five chapters, we will introduce the field of *inferential statistics*, which will enable us to start to make generalizations about unmeasured *populations* based upon our measured *sample*. The relationship between descriptive and inferential statistics is illustrated in Fig. 4.1, which is reproduced here from Fig. 1.1 for convenience. On the left is the population data, about which we do not have full knowledge. We only have knowledge of a measured subset of the population, which we term the sample. Descriptive statistics is used to describe and summarize this sample. Inferential statistics gets its name because we attempt to "infer", "deduce", or reach "conclusions" about the population using just information from the sample gathered.

For instance, consider the example we introduced in Chapter 1 of estimating the average height of first-year undergraduate students. To compute the correct answer, we would need to measure the height of every first-year undergradu-

Statistics for Biomedical Engineers and Scientists. https://doi.org/10.1016/B978-0-08-102939-8.00013-X

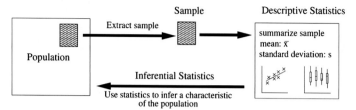

FIGURE 4.1

Overview of how population and sample are related, and the roles of descriptive and inferential statistics.

ate in the country, which is clearly not practical. However, if we measure the height of a large enough sample of the population we may be able to make a good enough guess at what the actual average height is. To be able to make such an inference, we *need the sample to be a random and representative subset of the population*. If this assumption is incorrect, then our deductions may be false. For instance, suppose that we chose as our sample all first-year under-graduate students from a college that awarded lots of basketball scholarships – clearly this may lead to an inaccurate estimate of the population height be-cause basketball players are likely to be of above average height, so our sample is not representative of the population. Ensuring that our sample is random and representative of our population can require careful experimental design (see Chapter 9).

4.2 NOTATION

The following notation will be used to discriminate between sample and pop-ulation values in this and subsequent chapters:

- $\bar{x}$: sample mean
- s: sample standard deviation
- μ: population mean
- σ: population standard deviation

For example, returning to our average heights example, μ and σ would repre-sent the actual mean and standard deviation of the heights of the population of first-year undergraduates, whereas $\bar{x}$ and s would represent the mean and standard deviation of our random sample.

4.3 PROBABILITY

As stated before, in inferential statistics we try to draw conclusions, or infer-ences, about the population based upon a sample. Because the sample is neces-sarily incomplete such conclusions are subject to some uncertainty. Therefore we begin this chapter with a brief overview of probability theory, which can be used to compute and express uncertainty.

4.3.1 Probabilities of Single Events

The word probability can be defined as "the chance of an event occurring". For example, suppose that we have a bag containing 10 balls, 5 white and 5 black, and we take one ball from the bag at random. The probability of taking a white ball is 0.5, or 1 in 2. Similarly, the probability of taking a black ball is 0.5. If the bag contained 4 white balls and 6 black balls, then the probabilities become 0.4 and 0.6, respectively. Note that in both cases the sum of the two probabilities was 1. This is true generally in probability: all probabilities should have a value between 0 and 1, and the sum of the probabilities for all possible outcomes should be 1.

Now let us introduce some terminology regarding probabilities:

- A *trial* is an action that results in one of several possible *outcomes* (e.g. taking a ball from the bag can result in one of 10 possible outcomes, one for each ball).
- An *experiment* is a series of trials (e.g. taking several balls from the bag).
- An *event* is a collection of specific outcomes that have something in common (e.g. the event of taking a white ball from the bag corresponds to 5 possible outcomes if there are 5 white balls).

Linking this back to the idea of a population and a sample, we can think of a trial as being like drawing a single value from a population and of an experiment as drawing a sample of several such values.

There are two ways of determining probability values: the *a priori* definition and the *relative frequency* definition. The a priori definition can be used only in the special case of *equally likely outcomes*. For example, when rolling a die, there are six possible outcomes: 1, 2, 3, 4, 5, and 6. If the die is unbiased, then we can assume that all of these outcomes are equally likely. Similarly, we can say that the chances of getting an even or an odd number are equally likely, since both *events* consist of three possible *outcomes*.

We can now give an a priori definition of probability: if an experiment has n equally likely outcomes and r of the outcomes are in the event E, then the probability $P(E)$ of E is r/n. So for the event of rolling an odd number with a die, there are $n = 6$ possible outcomes, the event E consists of $r = 3$ outcomes in which the die rolled an odd (1, 3, 5) number, and so $P(E) = 3/6 = 0.5$.

Now let us consider another example: the chance of you winning the Nobel prize. Again, we have two possible outcomes, yes and no. Can we use the a priori definition of probability here? If we do, then the chance of you winning the Nobel prize is 1/2, or 0.5. Unless you are extremely clever, this is not the true probability. The reason for this mistake is that the two outcomes are not equally likely: the chance of you not winning the Nobel prize is, unfortunately, much higher than the chance of you winning it. In such cases, we must use an alternative means to estimate the probability: the *relative frequency* definition. This involves performing an experiment to gather data about different events and then making an estimate of the probabilities based on the events observed. Specifically, if we perform n trials and r of them result in an event E, then we estimate the probability of E occurring as $P(E) = r/n$. If the number of trials is large enough, then the computed probability will be a reasonable approximation of the true probability. So, to return to the Nobel prize example, we could take a random sample of the world's population and find out how many of them have won a Nobel prize. Obviously, as the chance of winning a Nobel prize is quite small, we would need to take a very large sample, but if it is large enough, then our estimated probability should be accurate.[1]

4.3.2 Probabilities of Multiple Events

So far we have dealt only with single events. However, in many real-world situations we will be interested in probabilities of multiple events. In such cases, there are two laws that we need to be aware of, the *multiplication law* and the *addition law*.

Multiplication Law

The multiplication law defines the probability of two events *both* occurring. Therefore, in logical terms it deals with the *AND* operator (which is often denoted by the symbol $\wedge$). The general form for the multiplication law for two events A and B is

$$P(A \wedge B) = P(A)P(B|A), \tag{4.1}$$

where $P(B|A)$ denotes the probability of B occurring *given that A has occurred* (this is known as a *conditional probability*).

For instance, consider the example of drawing random cards from a pack of 52 playing cards. We will draw two cards from the pack without replacing the first card. We will denote by A the chance of drawing an ace for the first card and by B the chance of drawing an ace for the second card. What is the probability of drawing two aces, that is, $P(A \wedge B)$? For the first card, we know that there are 52 cards and 4 aces. All of the outcomes are equally likely, so using the a priori definition of probability, the chance of drawing an ace is $P(A) = 4/52 = 0.077$. When drawing the second card, there are 51 remaining cards, but the number of aces will depend upon the result of the first draw. In other words, $P(B|A)$

---

[1]In fact, in this example there would be no difficulty in using the entire population as the sample since it is quite easy to find out how many living Nobel prize winners there are, and we can also find out the population of the Earth. This will not always be the case though.

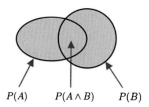

$P(A)$ $P(A \wedge B)$ $P(B)$

FIGURE 4.2
Venn diagram illustrating the relationship between $P(A)$, $P(B)$, and $P(A \wedge B)$. The ellipse is $P(A)$, the circle is $P(B)$, and the intersection of the ellipse and the circle is $P(A \wedge B)$. The gray-shaded area represents $P(A \vee B)$ and can be computed as the sum of $P(A)$ and $P(B)$ minus $P(A \wedge B)$.

is *not* equal to $P(B|\neg A)$ ($\neg$ is the symbol for the logical *NOT* operator). According to Eq. (4.1), we need to calculate $P(B|A)$. Given that the first card was an ace, there are only 3 aces left in the pack of 51, so $P(B|A) = 3/51 = 0.0588$. Therefore we can compute $P(A \wedge B)$ as the product of 0.077 and 0.0588, which is 0.0045.

Now suppose that we repeat the previous experiment, but this time we replace the first card before drawing the second one. In this case the result of the first draw has no influence on the result of the second draw: the chance of getting an ace on the second draw will always be $4/52 = 0.077$. In probability, we say that the events A and B are *statistically independent*. If A and B are statistically independent, then we can rewrite Eq. (4.1) in a simpler form:

$$P(A \wedge B) = P(A)P(B). \tag{4.2}$$

Generally, we can say that if A and B are statistically independent, then $P(B|A) = P(B)$.

Addition Law

The second way of combining probabilities is the *addition law*. This defines the probability of *either* of two events, or *both*, occurring. Therefore, in logical terms it deals with the *OR* operator (denoted by $\vee$). The general form of the addition law is

$$P(A \vee B) = P(A) + P(B) - P(A \wedge B). \tag{4.3}$$

At first, subtracting $P(A \wedge B)$ in Eq. (4.3) may seem strange. But consider Fig. 4.2. This shows the two probabilities $P(A)$ and $P(B)$ represented by an ellipse and a circle. What we want to compute, $P(A \vee B)$, corresponds to the shaded area. If we simply added $P(A)$ and $P(B)$, then we would end up including the intersection of the ellipse and the circle twice. This intersection represents $P(A \wedge B)$, so therefore this term must be subtracted to compute $P(A \vee B)$.

As with the multiplication law, we can identify a special case for the addition law in which the equation can be rewritten more simply. This special case relates to *mutually exclusive* events. Two events are mutually exclusive if they cannot both occur, that is, there would be no intersection in Fig. 4.2. In the playing cards example, it is possible that an ace will be drawn both times, that is, A and B will both occur, and therefore they are not mutually exclusive. But consider the example of probabilities of students on a particular degree programme getting different classifications for their degree (i.e. 1st, upper 2nd, lower 2nd, or 3rd). We denote these probabilities by $P(A)$, $P(B)$, $P(C)$, and $P(D)$, respectively. Now suppose that we wish to compute the probability of a randomly selected student from the programme gaining either a 1st or an upper 2nd. In this case, we can write

$$P(A \vee B) = P(A) + P(B) \tag{4.4}$$

since the chance of the student gaining both a 1st *and* an upper 2nd (i.e. $P(A \wedge B)$) is zero. In other words, A and B are mutually exclusive events.

■ Activity 4.1

O4.B

A hospital data analysis team wants to analyze the chances of success/failure in a particular type of surgery based upon whether or not the patients had prior risk factors. The risk factors they initially want to consider are *hypertension* (high blood pressure) and *prehypertension* (slightly high blood pressure, with an increased risk of developing hypertension). The following data have been gathered.

Risk factor	Success	Failure	Totals
Hypertension	10	7	17
Prehypertension	6	4	10
Neither	59	14	73
Totals	75	25	100

Answer the following questions about the data:

1. What is the probability that a randomly selected patient has hypertension?
2. From the table, what is the probability that a randomly selected patient has both hypertension and had failed surgery?
3. Compute the same probability as in the previous part using the multiplication rule.
4. Are having hypertension and having prehypertension mutually exclusive?
5. What is the probability that a randomly selected patient with neither hypertension nor pre-hypertension had failed surgery?

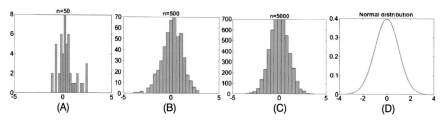

FIGURE 4.3

How a probability distribution function and histograms are related. The figure shows how, as the sample size increases, the histogram tends towards the probability distribution function. The images show histograms of samples from a normally distributed population with: (A) size 50; (B) size 500; (C) size 5000; and (D) the corresponding probability distribution function.

6. What is the probability that a randomly selected patient either has pre-hypertension or had successful surgery?

4.4 PROBABILITY DISTRIBUTIONS

Now that we have seen what probabilities are and how they can be calculated, let us look at the concept of *probability distributions*. In inferential statistics, we often make assumptions about the way the underlying population data are distributed. A *probability distribution* can be thought of as a continuous histogram of the entire population, as shown in Fig. 4.3. A distribution specifies the probability for each possible outcome of an experiment. Probability distribution functions are normalized so that the area underneath the curve equals one. Note also that in Fig. 4.3 the probability distribution function is *continuous* rather than discrete as in the probability examples given above, but the same concepts can be applied to both discrete and continuous data.

If we can reasonably assume that our sample data come from a particular type of probability distribution, then we can use this information to perform more powerful statistical analyses on our sample data. This approach is known as *parametric* hypothesis testing, and we will cover these techniques in Chapter 5. The alternative approach is *nonparametric* hypothesis testing, which we will cover in Chapter 6.

There are many types of continuous distribution used in statistical analyses, for example, uniform, exponential, gamma, and so on (see Fig. 4.4 for some examples). But by far the most commonly encountered distribution is the *normal* distribution, which is shown in Fig. 4.4C and which we already briefly saw in Section 2.4.2.

4.4.1 The Normal Distribution

The normal distribution is important because a large number of natural processes produce data that approximately fit to a normal distribution. We will

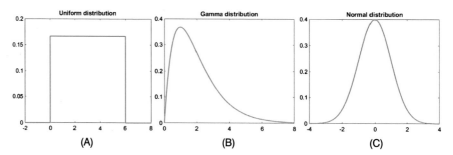

FIGURE 4.4

Example probability distributions: (A) uniform distribution; (B) gamma distribution; (C) normal distribution.

explain in the next section exactly why this is, but there are many examples of natural quantities that are approximately normally distributed, for example heights, weights, IQs, and so on.

The normal distribution was first described in 1809 by Carl Friedrich Gauss,[2] hence its alternative name, the *Gaussian* distribution. The equation describing the distribution for a random variable x is

$$N(x, \mu, \sigma) = \frac{1}{\sqrt{2\pi\sigma^2}} e^{\frac{(x-\mu)^2}{2\sigma^2}}, \tag{4.5}$$

where μ is the mean of the distribution, and σ its standard deviation. By a *random variable* we simply mean some variable or quantity whose value is random (but is determined by some probability distribution).

The mean μ determines the position along the x-axis of the peak of the distribution, whilst the standard deviation σ determines how "spread out" the distribution is: for a larger σ, the distribution will be "flatter" and have longer "tails" (i.e. the ends of the distribution will go on for longer). Some examples of normal distributions with different standard deviations are shown in Fig. 4.5A.

The area under a normal distribution is always equal to 1, regardless of its standard deviation. This is a useful property because we know from Section 4.3.1 that the probabilities of all outcomes should sum to 1. Furthermore, based upon Eq. (4.5) it is possible to compute what proportions of the total area under the distribution curve lie within certain distances (as multiples of the standard deviation) from the mean. These proportions are shown in Fig. 4.5B, and they will become important later on in this chapter.

The normal distribution is very important in inferential statistics because it is closely linked to the most important piece of theory underpinning parametric hypothesis testing, the *central limit theorem*.

---

[2] See Chapter 7's *Famous Statistician*.

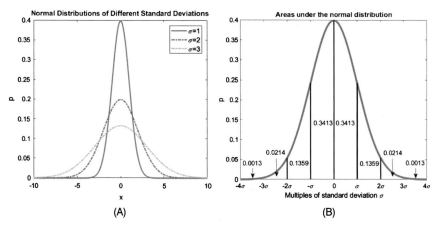

FIGURE 4.5

The normal distribution: (A) normal distributions with mean zero and different standard deviations σ; (B) areas under the normal distribution curve within multiples of the standard deviation.

4.5 WHY THE NORMAL DISTRIBUTION IS SO IMPORTANT: THE CENTRAL LIMIT THEOREM

The *central limit theorem* is a key concept in understanding the field of parametric hypothesis testing. The theorem explains why the normal distribution appears so regularly in nature. It deals with samples taken from a population of *statistically independent* random variables (i.e. the occurrence of one does not affect the occurrence of another; see Section 4.3.2). This is the case for most statistical data that we analyze, for example, one person's height does not depend on how tall somebody else is. Therefore, the theorem is widely applicable in statistical analysis, and furthermore it has important implications for how we can go about inferring conclusions about the population from the sample data. We first state in simple terms what the theorem says and then review its implications.

■ **Central Limit Theorem**

The central limit theorem states that, even if a population probability distribution is not normal, the distribution of mean values of samples from the distribution will be approximately normal for large enough sample sizes. ■

Let us first consider exactly what this is telling us. All population variables have an associated probability distribution. This distribution specifies what the chances are of getting each possible value of the variable if we were to choose a random subject from the population. For example, for the population of heights of first-year undergraduates, what would be the probability of a particular height if we randomly chose a first-year undergraduate student?

Now suppose that, instead of choosing one person, we choose several people and average their heights. This gives us a single value. If we were to repeat this process multiple times, then we would get a number of mean height values. *These mean height values would themselves have an associated probability distribution.* The central limit theorem is telling us that it does not matter how strange or non-normal the *original* population distribution was (i.e. of individual values such as heights) – the distribution of mean values will always be approximately normal so long as the sample size (i.e. how many values we compute the mean from) is large enough. This may seem surprising at first, so to convince ourselves, let us consider Fig. 4.6. Fig. 4.6A shows a histogram of 10,000 values randomly sampled from a uniform probability distribution. As we would expect, it looks uniform, and not even close to being normal. Fig. 4.6B shows what happens if we sample two values at a time and compute their mean (this is still a histogram of 10,000 values, but they are all mean values). Figs. 4.6C and 4.6D show the histograms produced by sampling 3 and 30 values at a time, respectively. Note that the larger the sample size, the closer the distribution of mean values gets to a normal distribution.

How close we get to a normal distribution depends upon the underlying population distribution and the number of values sampled, the sample size. If the original population distribution was close to normal, then we do not need large sample sizes for the distribution of means to also be approximately normal. If the original distribution was far from normal, we will need larger sample sizes for the distribution of means to become close to normal. As a rule-of-thumb, for most underlying population distributions, sample sizes of 30 or more are usually sufficient to get close to a normal distribution of mean values.

The theorem explains why the normal distribution appears so frequently in nature. Many natural quantities are the result of several independent processes. For example, our height may be influenced by our genetic make-up, our diet and our lifestyle, amongst other things. So we can think of the final quantity (height) as being in some sense the "average" of all of these influences. The central limit theorem tells us that if there are enough influencing factors, then the final quantity will be approximately normally distributed. This fact has the important implication that we can often make the assumption of normality in population distributions, and this allows us to apply parametric statistical methods to make stronger inferences about our data.

4.6   STANDARD ERROR OF THE MEAN

We now know that the population of mean values computed from sample data can often be assumed to be normally distributed. But what else can we say about its distribution? Can we say anything about how spread out the distribution will be (i.e. its standard deviation)? In statistics, we refer to this standard deviation (i.e. of mean values) as the *standard error of the mean*.

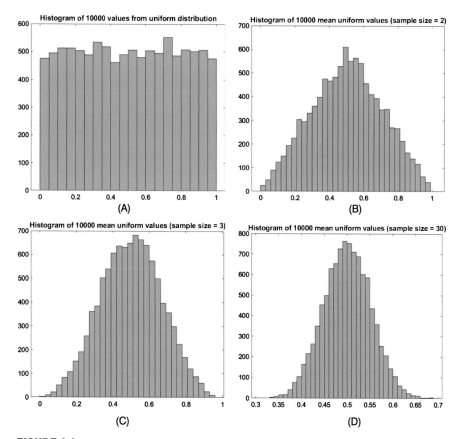

FIGURE 4.6
Demonstration of the central limit theorem – computing means of random samples from a uniform distribution with different sample sizes: (A) shows no averaging, just a histogram of the values of 10,000 samples of size 1 (i.e. single values) from the uniform distribution; (B) shows the histogram of mean values obtained by averaging 2 values from the uniform distribution; (C) averaging 3 values; (D) averaging 30 values. Note how the histograms become closer to a normal distribution as the number of values used to calculate the mean increases.

The formula for the standard error of the mean can be derived using knowledge of how to determine the variance of a sum of independent random variables. First, we denote by $x_1, \ldots, x_n$ a sample of n values (i.e. random variables) from a population with mean μ and standard deviation σ. The variance of the population is simply σ^2 (the variance is the square of the standard deviation; see Section 1.5.1), and it can be shown that the variance of $x_1 + x_2 + \ldots + x_n$ is $n\sigma^2$. Therefore, the variance of $\frac{x_1 + x_2 + \cdots + x_n}{n}$ (i.e. the sample mean) is $\frac{1}{n^2} n\sigma^2 = \frac{\sigma^2}{n}$. The standard deviation of the sample mean is simply the square root of this, $\frac{\sigma}{\sqrt{n}}$. Now, assuming that our sample standard deviation s is a good estimate of our population standard deviation σ, we have the equation for the standard

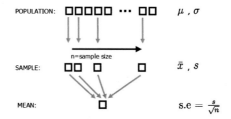

FIGURE 4.7
The relationship between the population, the sample, the mean of the sample and the standard error of the mean (s.e.).

error of the mean (s.e.) based only on information about our sample:

$$s.e. = \frac{s}{\sqrt{n}}, \tag{4.6}$$

where s is the calculated standard deviation of the sample, and n is the sample size. Note that the assumption that $s = \sigma$ will be true so long as n is large, typically more than 30. We are also assuming that the mean value $\bar{x}$ is drawn from a normal distribution (which we know from the central limit theorem is true for large n).

To summarize, the relationship between the population mean and standard deviation, the sample mean and standard deviation, and the standard error of the mean is illustrated in Fig. 4.7: the population mean and standard deviation are denoted by μ and σ; the mean and standard deviation of a sample x drawn from the population are $\bar{x}$ and s; and the standard error is the spread of the distribution of these mean values.

Note the following points about the standard error:

- It increases with s: if our sample data have lots of variation, then we are less certain about the mean value that we calculate.
- It decreases with $\sqrt{n}$: if we have more data, then we are more confident about the values we calculate, but note the diminishing returns due to the square root. If we currently have $n = 25$, then to be twice as confident in our mean value calculation, we would have to increase n by a factor of 4 to $n = 100$.
- The units of the standard error are the same as the units of the original data.

Going back to the first-year undergraduate student heights example from Chapter 1, the sample mean was $\bar{x} = 168.3$ cm, the sample standard deviation was $s = 9.1$ cm, and the sample size was $n = 40$. Therefore the standard error of the mean is s.e. $= \frac{9.1}{\sqrt{40}} = 1.44$ cm. This would often be written as "the mean height in the class was 168.3 ± 1.44 cm (1 s.e., $n = 40$)", where the details in brackets tell the reader which unreliability measure has been used and the sample size. Standard errors are often used as error bars in visualizations (see Section 1.6.1).

■ **Activity 4.2**

The birth weights of 100 babies were measured and recorded from a ran-   *O4.D*
dom sample of births at a hospital. The mean and standard deviation of the
weights were 3.7 kg and 1.0 kg, respectively.

1. If another 100 weights were recorded from a new random sample from the same hospital, what is the approximate probability that their mean will lie between 3.5 kg and 3.9 kg?
2. How many weights would need to be measured to be twice as confi-dent of the mean weight value?

                                                                         ■

4.7 CONFIDENCE INTERVALS OF THE MEAN

Confidence intervals are another way of expressing the reliability of our esti-mated mean value, and they build on the concept of the standard error of the mean that we introduced in the previous section. For now, we can think of a confidence interval as defining some range of values for a variable that repre-sent how confident we are about our estimated mean value for it (we will come to a more strict definition later). If we are less confident about the value of our mean, then it will have a larger confidence interval. If we are more confident, then it will have a smaller confidence interval. We can specify a degree of con-fidence that we would like to achieve: a standard degree is a 95% confidence interval, but if we would like to be more confident, then we could report a 99% confidence interval, in which case the interval reported will be larger. If we wanted to be 100% confident, then (as nothing is certain in statistics) the interval would have to be infinitely wide.

For example, suppose that we have taken a sample (of size $n > 30$) from a pop-ulation, and we have calculated the mean value $\bar{x}$. What can we say about the likely error in this mean value? From the central limit theorem we know that mean values have a normal distribution. We also know the standard deviation of the distribution, which is the standard error of the mean $\frac{s}{\sqrt{n}}$. Therefore we can produce a plot of the distribution around our sample mean – this will look like Fig. 4.5, but it would be centered on the sample mean $\bar{x}$. This distribution is telling us the likelihood of different values for subsequent estimates of the mean (from different samples). Based upon the properties of the normal dis-tribution shown in Fig. 4.5, we can work out a range of values within which a certain percentage of subsequent estimates of the mean will lie. For example, we can say that 68.3% ($=100\% \times (0.3413 + 0.3413)$) of such estimates would

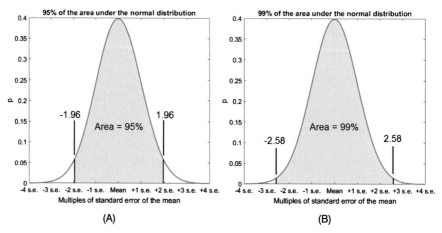

FIGURE 4.8
How far from the mean value do we need to go so that the area under the normal distribution curve is 95% or 99% of the total area under the curve? The answers are: (A) 1.96 standard deviations (i.e. standard errors) for 95% and (B) 2.58 standard deviations (standard errors) for 99%.

lie within one standard error from our current estimate of the mean. Similarly, 95.4% ($=100\% \times (0.3413 + 0.3413 + 0.1359 + 0.1359)$) would lie within two standard errors of the mean.

We can also turn these calculations around and ask: what range of mean values would we expect to find 95% of the time? This range can be calculated from Eq. (4.5) and turns out to be plus or minus 1.96 standard deviations (i.e. standard errors of the mean), as shown in Fig. 4.8A. For 99%, the figure is plus or minus 2.58 standard deviations (see Fig. 4.8B). This range of values for a given degree of confidence represents our confidence interval.

As an example of calculating confidence intervals, let us go back to our student heights example. Based upon our calculated standard error of the mean of 1.44 cm, we can now say that our 95% confidence interval is between 165.48 cm and 171.12 cm (i.e. $168.3 - 1.96 \cdot 1.44$ and $168.3 + 1.96 \cdot 1.44$). Our 99% confidence interval is between 164.58 cm and 172.02 cm (i.e. $168.3 - 2.58 \cdot 1.44$ and $168.3 + 2.58 \cdot 1.44$). Note that the above values (1.96 and 2.58) can only be used if the sample size is reasonably large ($n > 30$), meaning that the distribution of means is normal. For smaller sample sizes, values computed from the Student's t-distribution should be used. This will be covered in Section 5.5.

Finally, note that a strict definition of a confidence interval of the mean (e.g. for 95% confidence) is that if we were to compute many such confidence intervals from different samples, the proportion of them that contain the true population mean would tend towards 95%. Note that this is *not* the same as saying that there is a 95% chance that the population mean lies within a single confidence interval. Once we have computed a confidence interval, the population mean either lies within it or it does not, and no probabilities are necessary.

■ **Activity 4.3**

In this activity, we continue with the example of estimating babies' weights that we introduced in Activity 4.2. Recall that 100 babies were weighed and the mean and standard deviation of their weights were 3.7 kg and 1.0 kg, respectively.

O4.E

Compute both 95% and 99% confidence intervals of the mean weight value.   ■

4.8 SUMMARY

Inferential statistics deals with the process of inferring information about a population based on a sample from that population. Because the sample size is typically significantly smaller than the size of the population, such inferred information is subject to a measure of uncertainty.

Probabilities define the chance of an event occurring. Probability distributions are continuous histograms of the entire population – they define the probabilities of a variable taking any given value. Common probability distributions are the normal distribution, the uniform distribution, and the gamma distribution.

The central limit theorem states that the distribution of means determined from samples from a population always has an approximately normal distribution, so long as the sample size is large enough. This theorem is important in the field of inferential statistics because it allows us to define measures of reliability for statistics computed from samples.

Two such reliability measures were introduced in this chapter, the standard error of the mean and confidence intervals of the mean. The standard error of the mean is the standard deviation of mean values computed from samples from a population. Confidence intervals can be computed using the standard error of the mean and knowledge of the area under a normal distribution.

4.9 PROBABILITY DISTRIBUTIONS AND MEASURES OF RELIABILITY USING MATLAB

4.9.1 Probability Distributions

There are many built-in functions in MATLAB for performing different types of operations with probability distributions. For example, random numbers can be sampled from distributions using the following commands:

```
y = rand(m,n)
```

Creates an m × n array of random values sampled from a *uniform* distribution between 0 and 1:

```
y = randn(m,n)
```

Creates an m × n array of random values from the *standard normal distribution.* The standard normal distribution has $\mu = 0$ and $\sigma = 1$.

```
y = gamrnd(a, b, m, n)
```

Creates an m × n array of random values sampled from a *gamma* distribution with shape parameter a and scale parameter b.

In addition, the following functions enable specific types of calculation using the normal distribution:

```
y = normpdf(x, m, s)
```

Compute the value of the normal distribution with mean m and standard deviation s at points x:

```
p = normcdf(x, m, s)
```

Computes the value of the normal *cumulative distribution function* at value(s) x. The cumulative distribution function represents the total area under the normal distribution from *–infinity* to x. The arguments m and s are the mean and standard deviation, respectively, of the normal distribution.

```
x = norminv(p, m, s)
```

Computes the value of the *inverse* normal cumulative distribution function at value(s) p. The inverse cumulative distribution function takes a proportion p and returns the value x that has that proportion of the curve between it and *–infinity*. The arguments m and s are the mean and standard deviation, respectively, of the normal distribution.

4.9.2 Standard Error of the Mean

There is no built-in function in MATLAB for computing the standard error of the mean, but the calculations involved are straightforward as the following code illustrates:

```
n = 10; % sample size
x = randn(n,1); % sample from standard normal distribution
se = std(x)/sqrt(n); % compute standard error of mean
```

4.9.3 Confidence Interval of the Mean

The standard error of the mean can be used to compute confidence intervals of the mean as follows:

```
% compute standard error of the mean as before
n = 10; % sample size
x = randn(n,1); % sample from standard normal distribution
se = std(x)/sqrt(n); % standard error of mean

% compute 95%/99% confidence intervals
m = mean(x);
ci95 = [m-1.96*se, m+1.96*se];
ci99 = [m-2.58*se, m+2.58*se];
```

4.10   FURTHER RESOURCES

■ A nice tutorial on the central limit theorem can be found here:
   http://www.statisticshowto.com/probability-and-statistics/
   normal-distributions/central-limit-theorem-definition-examples/

4.11   EXERCISES

Perform the following tasks, either by hand or using MATLAB, as specified:

■ **Exercise 4.1**

The blood groups of 250 volunteers (131 male, 119 female) were determined   *O4.B*
using blood tests: 62 had type A, 70 had type B, 83 had type O, and 35 had
type AB. Answer the following questions by hand.

1. Are the blood types mutually exclusive?
2. If a volunteer is selected at random, what is the probability that they
    have blood type AB?
3. If a volunteer is selected at random, what is the probability that they
    have either blood type A or B?
4. Assuming that gender and blood type are statistically independent,
    what is the probability that a randomly selected volunteer is a female
    with blood type O?

                                                                        ■

■ **Exercise 4.2**

A biomedical engineering company manufacture artificial hip joints from ti-   *O4.D, O4.E*
tanium alloy. The femoral head for the joint needs to be precision machined
to fit the corresponding socket in the pelvis. To test their manufacturing
process, the company have produced 25 femoral heads with an intended
diameter of 45 mm. The femoral heads were measured, and their mean and
standard deviation were found to be 45.1 mm and 0.5 mm, respectively.

1. Calculate the standard error of the mean by hand.

2. If another 25 femoral heads were produced, what is the probability that their mean diameter would be within 0.1 mm of the target value of 45 mm? Work out the answer by hand.
3. Calculate both 95% and 99% confidence intervals of the mean femoral head diameter by hand and then verify your results using MATLAB. ■

■ Exercise 4.3

O4.C   In this exercise, you will experimentally verify the central limit theorem. Perform these tasks using MATLAB:

1. Write code to compute the means of a number of samples of a given size from a uniform distribution. Compute 1000 mean values and plot a histogram of them. Perform this experiment using samples of size 1, 2, 5 and 30.
2. Repeat the experiments using a normal distribution rather than a uniform distribution.
3. Repeat the experiments using a gamma distribution with shape parameter 3 and scale parameter 2. ■

■ Exercise 4.4

O4.D, O4.E   A research programme is looking to investigate a new treatment for heart failure patients. One possible indicator that is being investigated to quantify the success of the treatment is the left ventricular end systolic volume (LVESV). LVESV can be measured using magnetic resonance imaging (MRI) or ultrasound imaging, and decreased LVESV can be a sign of improved heart function. Pre-treatment LVESV data (in mL) have been collected from 10 heart failure patients who underwent the new treatment. The LVESV values are contained in the file "lvesv_pre.txt", which is available from the book's web site.

Use MATLAB to perform the following tasks.

1. Compute the mean and standard error of the mean of the LVESV data.
2. Assuming that the distribution of mean values is normal, compute 95% and 99% confidence intervals of the mean LVESV.

Data were also collected from the same patients after treatment. These data are contained in the file "lvesv_post.txt". A decrease in LVESV may be evidence of successful treatment.

3. Compute the differences between the LVESV data pre- and post-treatment.

4. Compute the mean of the differences and the 95% confidence interval of the mean difference.
5. Does the confidence interval contain the value 0? What does this tell us about the chance that the treatment decreases LVESV?

Exercise 4.5

Write MATLAB code to "empirically" (i.e. experimentally) estimate the standard deviation of the distribution of mean values and compare this to the standard error of the mean computed from a single sample using Eq. (4.6). These two values should be approximately the same. In other words, for the empirical estimate, generate a large number of samples of a specified size, compute mean values for each one, and then compute the standard deviation of these means.

O4.D

Exercise 4.6

Use MATLAB to determine how often you would expect a random value taken from a normal distribution to fall within 1.15 standard deviations of the mean of the distribution.

O4.C

Exercise 4.7

You already know the 1.96/2.58 figures for 95% and 99% confidence intervals. What is the corresponding figure for 50% confidence? In other words, within what multiple of the standard deviation will 50% of samples from a normal distribution fall? Use MATLAB to compute your answer.

O4.C, O4.D, O4.E

FAMOUS STATISTICIAN: PIERRE DE FERMAT

This chapter's Famous Statistician is not strictly speaking a statistician, but it is safe to say that much of modern statistics would not have been possible without him. Pierre de Fermat lived from 1601–1665 and was a French lawyer and amateur mathematician. He is one of the most famous mathematicians of all time and is probably best known for Fermat's last theorem, which was finally proved in 1995.

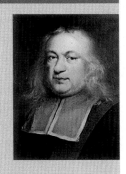

Fermat communicated most of his work in letters to friends, often with little or no proof of his theorems. He is regarded (along with his friend Blaise Pascal) as the founder of probability theory, which is the basis for much of modern statistics. The inspiration for probability theory apparently came from a friend of a friend of Fermat, who was a professional gambler. The gambler had been playing a game which had been interrupted before it was finished, and the players could not agree on a fair way to divide the pot. Fermat decided that the fairest way was to divide it according to each player's probability of winning at the point of interruption; for example, if a player had a 70% chance of winning, he should get 70% of the pot. As well as his work on probability theory, Fermat made significant and lasting contributions to the fields of number theory and analytic geometry.

CHAPTER 5

Inferential Statistics II: Parametric Hypothesis Testing

LEARNING OBJECTIVES

At the end of this chapter, you should be able to:

O5.A *Explain the general procedure for performing hypothesis tests and describe the types of error that can occur*

O5.B *Explain how the t-distribution differs from the normal distribution and how it can be useful when dealing with small samples*

O5.C *Compute confidence intervals for small samples by hand and using MATLAB*

O5.D *Choose and apply an appropriate Student's t-test by hand and using MATLAB, depending on whether there are one or two sets of sample data, and whether the data are paired or unpaired*

O5.E *Apply a z-test by hand and using MATLAB, to test if a sample comes from a distribution with known mean and variance*

5.1 INTRODUCTION

In the last chapter, we saw how knowledge of the normal distribution can be useful in making inferences about the nature of the population from sample data. This was possible because of the *central limit theorem*. Recall that the central limit theorem states that, given a population variable of interest, the distribution of mean values computed from samples of the variable will always be approximately normal regardless of the variable's population distribution. We also saw how the standard error and confidence intervals of the mean can be computed using knowledge of the distribution of mean values. In this chapter, we take this idea further and introduce ways in which specific hypotheses about the population can be tested.

5.2 HYPOTHESIS TESTING

A hypothesis test is a formal way of asking and answering a question about the population based upon sample data drawn from that population. As we

Statistics for Biomedical Engineers and Scientists. https://doi.org/10.1016/B978-0-08-102939-8.00014-1

typically do not have full access to the population data, any answer is subject to an element of uncertainty. Therefore it is normal to specify a *degree of confidence* that we wish to work to when doing hypothesis testing. For example, we may want to be 95% confident in the answer, or 99%. But remember that we can never be 100% confident in the answers that hypothesis tests provide.

Related to the degree of confidence is the concept of a *significance level*. A significance level of a hypothesis test is simply another way of stating the degree of confidence and is equal to one minus the degree of confidence expressed as a probability. So, if our degree of confidence is 95% (or 0.95 expressed as a probability), then our significance level is 0.05. The significance level is often denoted by α and is closely related to the concept of a *p-value*, which we will return to later in this chapter (see Section 5.5).

There are two different types of hypothesis test, *parametric* and *nonparametric*. Parametric hypothesis tests can be used if we can reasonably assume that our sample data come from a specific probability distribution. Nonparametric hypothesis tests are used when we cannot make this assumption; in other words, we have less knowledge about the population distribution of the variable we are testing. Parametric tests are preferred over nonparametric tests as they are usually more powerful.[1] In this chapter, we focus on parametric hypothesis tests.

When performing a hypothesis test, we are testing the validity of two different hypotheses about the data:

- *Null hypothesis*: "There is no difference in the population data, and so any apparent difference in the sample is due to random variation."
- *Alternative hypothesis*: "A real difference does exist, even though it may be partially obscured by random variations in the data."

The null hypothesis is effectively our default position. Unless we find evidence to the contrary, we will work on the assumption that it is true (although we can never actually be *sure* that it is true). The point of a hypothesis test is to try to demonstrate that the null hypothesis is false and instead the alternative hypothesis is true.

There are two types of error that can occur in hypothesis testing, which are connected to the two hypotheses:

---

[1]We will deal with concept of the *power* of a statistical test in Chapter 9, but for now just think of it as a measure of how likely the test is to succeed in finding a difference if there is one.

■ *Type I error*: Our hypothesis test finds a significant difference (and there-fore we reject the null hypothesis), but in reality there is no difference. These errors can be caused by choosing too low a degree of confidence (e.g. 90% rather than 95%).

■ *Type II error*: Our hypothesis test does not find any significant difference, and therefore we do not reject the null hypothesis, but in reality there is a difference (i.e. the alternative hypothesis is true). This can happen for a number of reasons, but most commonly it is due to not enough data being collected.

In this and subsequent chapters, we will see several different kinds of hypoth-esis test. But generally we will follow a standard sequence of activities. So the following checklist can be useful:

1. *Examine the data.*
2. *Formulate suitable null and alternative hypotheses, and choose a degree of con-fidence to work to.*
3. *Calculate a test statistic from the data.*
4. *Compare the test statistic with a critical value and decide if we can reject the null hypothesis.*

■ **Activity 5.1**

Are the following statements true or false?   *O5.A*

1. "A Type II error results in finding a difference when in reality no such difference exists."
2. "If we cannot reject the null hypothesis, then we accept it to be true."
3. "Choosing a high degree of confidence reduces the chance of a Type I error."

■

5.3 TYPES OF DATA FOR HYPOTHESIS TESTS

In this chapter, we review the most common parametric hypothesis tests for three specific cases based upon the type of data that we have:

■ One sample.
■ Two-sample paired data.
■ Two-sample unpaired data.

The *one-sample* case refers to when we have a single sample containing a num-ber of measurements of a variable. For example, the sample could contain the cholesterol levels of a sample of 20 patients. When we have a single sample, we typically want to use a parametric hypothesis test to compare the sample mean to a known value. To continue our cholesterol example, we may want to compare the sample mean to a normal healthy value of 5 mmol/L.

In other situations, we may have two samples of data, and then a typical question to ask is: "do the populations from which these two samples were drawn have different mean values?" We can identify two different cases for two sample data: *paired* data, in which there are one-to-one correspondences between the measurements in each sample, and *unpaired* data, in which there are no such correspondences. An example of paired two-sample data is if we took cholesterol measurements from the *same* group of patients before and after a treatment. The data are paired because we know which measurements correspond between the two samples (because they were taken from the same patient). An example of unpaired two-sample data is if we took cholesterol measurements from *two separate groups* of subjects, one from people who took a dietary supplement and the other who did not.

■ **Activity 5.2**

O5.D   What type of data do we have in the following scenarios? (i.e. one/two-sample, paired or unpaired)

1. We have measured the weights of two groups of subjects, one of which has an active lifestyle and the other of which has a sedentary lifestyle. We wish to know if the average weights of people with sedentary/active lifestyles are different.
2. We have used ultrasound imaging to estimate the ejection fractions (i.e. the percentage of blood pumped out of the left ventricle in each heart beat) of a group of heart patients. We wish to know if the values are different to a normal healthy value.
3. We have measured tumor size from Positron Emission Tomography (PET) imaging data acquired from a group of cancer patients. The patients underwent chemotherapy, and the tumor sizes were measured again. We wish to know if the tumors have changed size.

5.4   THE *t*-DISTRIBUTION AND STUDENT'S *t*-TEST

The most common type of parametric hypothesis test is the *Student's t-test*. This was developed by William Gosset,[2] who published under the pseudonym "Student". The test was specifically designed to work with smaller sample sizes. We saw in the last chapter that the central limit theorem states that the distribution of mean values is approximately normal for sufficiently large sample sizes

---

[2] See the Famous Statistician at the end of this chapter.

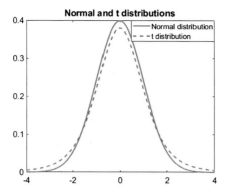

FIGURE 5.1

Comparison of t-distribution (dotted curve for a sample size $n = 6$) and normal distribution (solid curve). Note that the t-distribution has larger tails, that is, a greater probability of values far from the mean. The t-distribution will be slightly different for different values of n, and for large n, it will converge to the normal distribution.

(typically $n > 30$). One of Gosset's main contributions was to show that, for smaller sample sizes, the distribution of mean values follows the t-distribution, an example of which is shown in Fig. 5.1.

Versions of the Student's t-test allow us to test whether the mean of the population from which our sample was drawn differs from an expected value, or whether the means of two different populations differ. The test statistic of the t-test is known as the *t-value*. It is based on the standard error of the mean (see Section 4.6) and is of the general form

$$t = \frac{\text{difference to be tested}}{\text{standard error of the mean}}.$$

Note that, for all types of Student's t-test, it is assumed that the population variables of interest are approximately normally distributed. Furthermore, because the standard error of the mean is calculated using the sample standard deviation s, there is an additional assumption that the sample standard deviation is a good estimate of the population standard deviation σ. For normally distributed data, this is often a reasonable assumption.

5.5 ONE-SAMPLE STUDENT'S *t*-TEST

We will start off with the one-sample Student's t-test, which tests if the mean of the population from which our sample was drawn differs from an expected value. We will illustrate the test with a worked example. Professor A believes that she has devised a new method of producing the drug "Wonder" with much higher purity than has previously been possible. The government guidelines for drug purity state that the drug must have less than $\mu = 50$ contaminants. She

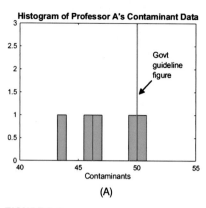
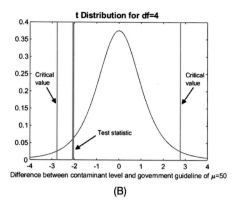

(A)   (B)

FIGURE 5.2

Professor A's one-sample t-test. (A) A histogram of the contaminant level in five drug batches produced by Professor A's researcher. The vertical line shows the government guideline contaminant level. (B) A t-distribution for $df = 4$. The symmetric vertical lines at ± 2.776 show the critical value required to be 95% sure that we can reject the null hypothesis. If we were to integrate the area under the curve outside of these two lines, then it would equal 5% of the total area. The third, thicker, vertical line at -2.053 shows the t-value calculated. As this line is inside the other two (i.e. $|t| < 2.776$), we cannot reject the null hypothesis.

sets her researcher to work to produce five batches of the drug. The researcher measures the contaminant values in each batch, resulting in the data (43.72 46.32 50.71 45.86 49.92). Based on these data, we can easily compute the sample mean and standard deviation: $\bar{x} = 47.31$, $s = 2.93$. Professor A would like to write a paper that states that her new method can produce the drug with a mean contaminant level lower than the government guideline of $\mu = 50$. Can Professor A publish based upon these results?

To answer this question, we will carry out a t-test. We will follow the checklist we introduced earlier, and so our first step is to examine the data. A histogram of Professor A's data is shown in Fig. 5.2A, which also shows the government guideline figure of $\mu = 50$. This is the expected mean value, which we will compare our data to. It is always worth visualizing the data in this way to get an impression of what the distribution is like and to spot any possible problems (e.g. outliers in the data). Here we do not see anything problematic, but we can see that there is one value above the guideline figure and four below.

Next, we form our hypotheses. The null hypothesis is that there is no difference between the population mean and 50. The alternative hypothesis is that there is such a difference. (Note that, at the moment, we are not asking if the mean is *less than* 50 as perhaps we should. We will come back to this point in Section 5.8.) We also need to choose a degree of confidence. For this test, we will work to 95% confidence, which corresponds to a significance level of $\alpha = 0.05$.

The next step is to calculate a test statistic. The equation for the test statistic for a one-sample Student's *t*-test is

$$t = \frac{\bar{x} - \mu}{s/\sqrt{n}}. \tag{5.1}$$

Recall that $\bar{x}$ is the sample mean, s is the standard deviation of the sample, n is the sample size, and $s/\sqrt{n}$ is the standard error of the mean (see Section 4.6). Therefore, for Professor A's data, we have $t = (47.31 - 50)/(2.93/\sqrt{5}) = -2.053$.

Now we need to find a critical value to compare our test statistic to. To do this, we need to determine the number of *degrees of freedom (df)* of the test. We can think of the degrees of freedom as being the number of unknowns (or independent variables) in the data that we are analyzing. This is clearly related to the sample size, but remember that we already know the mean value of the sample, so we can subtract one degree of freedom from the sample size n. Therefore, for a one-sample Student's *t*-test, there are $n - 1$ degrees of freedom. For our worked example, $n = 5$, so we have 4 degrees of freedom. We can then look up in a statistical table the critical value for a *t*-test with $\alpha = 0.05$ and $df = 4$. The table for this type of test is shown in Table A.1 in the Appendix. Based on this table, our critical *t* value is 2.776. For a one-sample Student's *t*-test, we can reject the null hypothesis if the absolute value of the calculated *t* statistic is greater than the critical value. The absolute value of our *t* statistic (i.e. 2.053) is less than the critical value of 2.776. Therefore, Professor A is *not* able to reject the null hypothesis at 95% confidence.

■ **The Intuition. Student's *t*-test**

Fig. 5.2B illustrates how this conclusion was reached. The curve shows a *t*-distribution for 4 degrees of freedom. This represents the distribution of the difference in mean contaminant level from the government guideline figure under the assumption that the null hypothesis is true, that is, the distribution is centered on zero, which means no difference between Professor A's contaminant levels and the guideline of $\mu = 50$. The horizontal axis represents the number of standard errors of the mean away from the actual mean (i.e. zero). 95% of the area under the curve is within the two thin vertical lines at ±2.776. Therefore, if the null hypothesis were true, there would be a less than 5% chance that our observed difference would be more than 2.776 standard errors of the mean away from zero. This probability would be low enough to reject the null hypothesis, that is, it would be less than the significance level. However, the observed difference (i.e. our test statistic $t = -2.053$) is shown as the bold vertical line, and it lies *between* the two lines at ±2.776. Therefore we *cannot* reject the null hypothesis in this case.

Note that the values in Table A.1 are simply precomputed values derived from the *t*-distribution curves for different degrees of freedom. That is, they simply state, for each curve (i.e. degrees of freedom), how many standard deviations away from the mean we would need to go so that the area under the curve was 90%/95%/99% (depending on the significance level). ■

The t-test (and many other tests) can return something known as a *p-value*. We came across the concept of a *p*-value in Section 2.4.1 in the context of correlation values. In the context of a Student's t-test, the p-value is essentially the probability that, *if the null hypothesis were true*, we would observe the kind of distribution (or a more unlikely one) that we have in our sample data just through random variation in the data. For this experiment, the p-value was 0.11, that is, 11% of the time results similar to or more extreme than those obtained by the researcher could just have occurred by chance if the null hypothesis were true. Again, this value can be derived from the properties of the t-distribution curve, that is, we could draw vertical lines at $\pm$ our test statistic and compute how much of the area under the curve lies beyond them. Professor A was aiming for a p-value below her significance level of 0.05, which would mean that there would be a less than 1 in 20 chance of seeing this type of data distribution purely by chance.

■ Activity 5.3

O5.A, O5.D

Cholesterol levels (in mmol/L) have been measured from 20 hospital patients. The mean and standard deviation of the measurements are 5.4 and 0.7, respectively. Use a one-sample Student's t-test to determine, with 99% confidence, whether the average cholesterol levels of the patients are significantly different from the normal healthy value of 5 mmol/L. ■

Returning to our worked example, Professor A is still confident in her new method and thinks that a Type II error (see Section 5.2) may have occurred. She decides that more data are needed, and so sets her researcher to work to produce five more batches of the drug using the new method. The results are (48.25 50.87 44.08 47.60 45.58). Combining these data with the previous batches gives an overall mean of $\bar{x} = 47.29$, $s = 2.61$, and $n = 10$. The histogram of these combined data is shown in Fig. 5.3A.

The calculated t-value from these data is -3.278. Our test statistic is now calculated with $n - 1 = 9$ degrees of freedom, and for $\alpha = 0.05$, the critical value from Table A.1 is 2.262. The absolute value of t is larger than this critical value, and so this time we can reject the null hypothesis and say that there *is* a significant difference between the mean contaminant level of the drug made using the new method and the government guidelines. The p-value was just 0.0096 and so below 1%. Therefore, there is less than a 1 in 100 chance of this type of data distribution (or a more extreme one) occurring due to random variation.

As this example shows, statistical significance can often be obtained, even if a difference is very small, by collecting more data (i.e. increasing n). How-

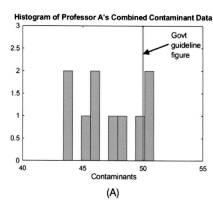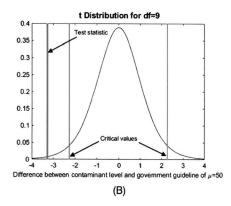

FIGURE 5.3

Professor A's one sample t-test using the new combined data. (A) A histogram of the contaminant level in 10 drug batches produced by the researcher. The vertical line shows the government guideline contaminant level. (B) A t-distribution for $df = 9$. The thin vertical lines at ± 2.262 show the critical value required to be 95% sure that we can reject the null hypothesis ($\alpha = 0.05$). If we were to integrate the area under the curve outside of these two lines it would equal 5% of the total area. The third, thicker, vertical line at -3.278 shows the t-value calculated. As this line is outside the other two (i.e. $|t| > 2.262$), we reject the null hypothesis.

ever, it is important to remember that *a statistically significant difference does not mean that the difference is important.* Whether or not the difference is important is determined by knowledge of the actual process being tested. For example, decreasing the contaminant level from 50 to 47 might have no effect on the users of the drug (as it is already almost pure, or the users are all insensitive to the contaminants). On the other hand, maybe there is a critical level of contaminant (e.g. at 48) above which there are serious side effects. These are all different questions, which need to be answered by further experimentation. All the statistical analysis from these data can tell us is whether the change in contaminant level is likely (or unlikely) to have happened by chance.

5.6 CONFIDENCE INTERVALS FOR SMALL SAMPLES

Before moving on to other types of hypothesis test, we now return briefly to the concept of confidence intervals that we introduced in Section 4.7. Those confidence interval values were computed using knowledge of the normal distribution, and as such they were valid only for relatively large sample sizes (>30 as a rough guide). Smaller sample sizes are very common due to time, cost, and/or ethical requirements. Means of smaller samples are *not* normally distributed, as we have just seen. But we also know that they can be approximated by the t-distribution. Therefore, to calculate confidence intervals for smaller samples, we can use the critical t-test values that were used earlier and are shown in Table A.1. Recall that these represent how many standard deviations (i.e. standard errors of the mean) away from the mean we would need

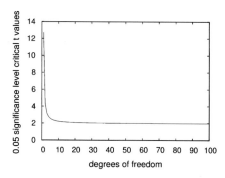

FIGURE 5.4

t-values for a 0.05 significance level as a function of the number of degrees of freedom.

to go to make the area under a *t*-distribution curve 90%/95%/99% (depending on the degree of confidence) of the total area. Fig. 5.4 shows how the critical *t*-value for $\alpha = 0.05$ changes as the number of degrees of freedom (i.e. the sample size) increases. The critical *t*-value rapidly decreases as the number of degrees of freedom increases from 1 to 10, and then it slowly approaches the normal distribution value of 1.96, which we used in the last chapter. This occurs because the *t*-distribution for large sample sizes is almost identical to a normal distribution.

Therefore, to calculate confidence intervals for small samples, we need to:

■ Decide which degree of confidence to work to (e.g. 95%, which equates to 0.05 significance).
■ Calculate the number of degrees of freedom, which is $n - 1$.
■ Look up the critical value of *t* from Table A.1.

Our confidence interval of the mean is then from

$$\bar{x} - \frac{ts}{\sqrt{n}} \quad \text{to} \quad \bar{x} + \frac{ts}{\sqrt{n}}. \tag{5.2}$$

Compare this equation to the way we calculated confidence intervals using the normal distribution in the last chapter: we added and subtracted a multiple of the standard error of the mean from the mean of the sample. For instance, for 95% confidence, we added/subtracted 1.96 times the standard error of the mean. In Eq. (5.2), we are simply adding and subtracting *t* times the standard error of the mean (i.e. $s/\sqrt{n}$). Therefore, as stated earlier, the critical *t*-values are telling us the multiples of the standard error of the mean that we need to use to include a certain percentage of the area under the *t*-distribution curve.

As a worked example of confidence intervals for small samples, we will again use the data about Professor A's new drug production technique. Professor A's

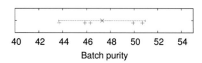

FIGURE 5.5

95% confidence interval and data points for the contaminant levels of the first five batches of the drug produced with the new method. The + symbols are the data points, the × symbol is the sample mean, and the dashed horizontal line represents the 95% confidence interval.

researcher initially produced five batches of the drug with the contaminant levels (43.72 46.32 50.71 45.86 49.92). The sample mean was $\bar{x} = 47.31$, and the sample standard deviation was $s = 2.93$. Therefore we follow the steps outlined before to compute confidence intervals:

- Decide which degree of confidence to work to; we will choose 95%, meaning a 0.05 significance level.
- Calculate the number of degrees of freedom, which is $n - 1 = 4$.
- Look up the critical value of t from Table A.1. For 0.05 significance and $df = 4$, this is 2.776.

We find that the 95% confidence interval of the mean for this sample of batches is between $47.31 - 2.776 \cdot 2.93/\sqrt{5}$ and $47.31 + 2.776 \cdot 2.93/\sqrt{5}$, that is, between 43.673 and 50.947. The original data and confidence interval are shown graphically in Fig. 5.5. The key point to note here is that the 95% confidence interval *includes* the value for the government guideline $\mu = 50$. Therefore from the confidence interval we *cannot* say that our mean value is likely (95% confidence) to be different from the government guideline figure. This is the same conclusion as our hypothesis test: Professor A was unable to reject the null hypothesis using these data. Both the confidence interval and the hypothesis test give the same result – it is just a different way of presenting the data.

We can also calculate the confidence interval for the data with 10 batches. The sample mean and standard deviation were $\bar{x} = 47.29$ and $s = 2.61$. With 9 degrees of freedom, the 0.05 significance level critical t-value is 2.262, and so the 95% confidence interval is now between $47.29 - 2.262 \cdot 2.61/\sqrt{10}$ and $47.29 + 2.262 \cdot 2.61/\sqrt{10}$, that is, between 45.42 and 49.16. This information is shown graphically in Fig. 5.6. Critically now the upper limit of the 95% confidence interval is *below* the government guideline value $\mu = 50$. This is another way of showing that we *can* now reject the null hypothesis and say that there is a significant difference between the contaminant levels of Professor A's method of producing the drug and $\mu = 50$. This is the same result as we achieved with the hypothesis test.

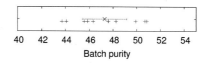

FIGURE 5.6

95% confidence interval and data points for the contaminant levels for ten batches of the drug produced with the new method. The + symbols are the data points, the × symbol is the sample mean, and the dashed horizontal line represents the 95% confidence interval.

■ Activity 5.4

O5.C

Wernicke–Korsakoff syndrome can be caused by a deficiency in vitamin B1 and is a known cause of dementia. A medical research project is investigating whether a vitamin B1 supplement can reduce the severity of the onset of dementia in patients with Wernicke–Korsakoff syndrome.

A cohort of 20 patients who have been diagnosed with Wernicke–Korsakoff syndrome were recruited onto the study. They were randomly divided into two groups of 10: a "test" group were given a weekly vitamin B1 supplement over the course of 6 months, and a "control" group received no medication.

The Mini Mental State Examination (MMSE) is a questionnaire that can be used to measure cognitive impairment. Subjects taking the questionnaire are given a score between 0 and 30, with lower scores representing more severe cognitive impairment.

The control and test groups each took the MMSE before starting the study and after 6 months. The recorded data were analyzed and found to be normally distributed. Summary statistics are shown in the table below, which shows the mean and standard deviation of the MMSE scores of the control and test groups before and after the 6-month trial period.

	Control		Test	
	Before	After	Before	After
Mean =	20.5	16.42	20.19	17.04
Std. dev. =	2.22	2.75	1.97	2.32

Compute 95% confidence intervals of the mean value for all four sets of data, that is, control group before and after and test group before and after. Comment on what the results tell you about the efficacy of the supplement.

■

5.7 TWO SAMPLE STUDENT'S *t*-TEST

Previously, we examined the use of the Student's *t*-test to calculate whether a mean of a population from which a sample was drawn and an expected value were different. A much more common situation is where we are comparing two samples, a test and a control sample. In this case the population mean is unknown. Instead, we are comparing two sample means $\bar{x}_t$ and $\bar{x}_c$ (the subscripts denote "test" and "control"). Now, as we are unsure of the accuracy of both mean values, it is a bit harder to achieve statistical significance. As described earlier in Section 5.3, we can identify two different situations where we have two samples of data, *paired data* and *unpaired data*. The Student's *t*-test works slightly differently for these two cases, and so we deal with each of these situations in separate sections below.

5.7.1 Paired Data

We start off by looking at a *t*-test using *paired data*. Recall that paired data occur when data values in the two samples correspond in some way, for example, data from the same people but at different times. We will illustrate the two-sample paired *t*-test using an example. A group of researchers want to test the efficacy of a new drug to treat hypertension (high blood pressure). End systolic blood pressure data (in mmHg) have been gathered from a group of eight patients suffering from mild to severe hypertension before treatment with the new drug and after treatment. We will call the pretreatment data the control data and the posttreatment data the test data. Our blood pressure measurements are:

Control:	175.4	188.3	147.4	178.6	173.2	156.9	165.7	173.4
Test:	152.3	159.7	155.7	166.2	149.1	162.3	163.5	146.0

Because the data were acquired from the same group of patients, it is considered to be *paired* data, that is, the blood pressure values for each patient before and after treatment are paired, or corresponding, as they were measured from the same subject. The basic procedure for a two-sample paired *t*-test is based on that for the one-sample *t*-test:

- Compute the *differences* between the paired sample data; then
- Perform a one-sample *t*-test on the difference data using an expected value μ of zero.

In other words, we test if the mean of the differences between the paired sample data is statistically significantly different from zero. We illustrate this using our hypertension example:

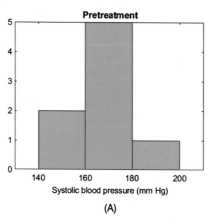
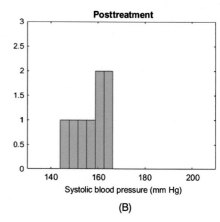

FIGURE 5.7

Histograms of the hypertension patient systolic blood pressure data: (A) pretreatment, (B) posttreatment.

■ Compute the differences. By subtracting the control values from the corresponding test values we get $(-23.1\ -28.6\ 8.3\ -12.4\ -24.1\ 5.4\ -2.2\ -27.4)$. From these differences we can compute the mean $\bar{d} = -13.0125$ and standard deviation $s_d = 15.0484$.

■ Perform a one-sample t-test using an expected value of zero. For this, we follow our checklist:

▦ *Examine the data*: See histograms in Fig. 5.7. We do not see any outliers, and by eye the posttreatment data seem lower.

▦ *Formulate hypotheses and choose degree of confidence*: Our null hypothesis is that there is no difference between the population means of the two variables, and our alternative hypothesis is that there is such a difference. We will work to 95% confidence.

▦ *Calculate a test statistic from the data*: Using Eq. (5.1), we compute $t = \frac{-13.0125}{15.0484/\sqrt{8}} = -2.4458$.

▦ *Compare the test statistic with a critical value and decide if we can reject the null hypothesis*: From Table A.1, for $df = n - 1 = 7$ and $\alpha = 0.05$, we have a critical t-value of 2.365. Because $|-2.4458| > 2.365$, we *can* reject the null hypothesis. This confirms our initial impression from examining the data.

Therefore, based on the sample data, we can conclude that taking the new drug results in a statistically significant difference in the end systolic blood pressure of the hypertension patients.

■ **Activity 5.5**

O5.D   A research project is investigating the use of machine learning to automatically derive biometric measurements from fetal ultrasound. One biometric of interest is head diameter. The machine learning based technique has been applied to a set of 20 fetal ultrasound images resulting in 20 head diameter estimates. An expert clinician has also manually measured the head diameter from the same set of images. The researchers would like to demonstrate that their technique can produce estimates of head diameter that are indistinguishable from those of the human expert.

The mean of the differences in head diameter between the machine learning based estimates and those of the human expert was 1.1 mm, and the standard deviation of the differences was 1.9 mm.

Perform a two-sample paired *t*-test to determine if the difference between the estimates made using the two approaches is significantly different to zero (99% confidence).   ◼

5.7.2 Unpaired Data

It is often the case that we do not have paired data to work with but we would still like to show statistical significance between two sets of data. To illustrate this case, we are going to continue with our example, in which Professor A has now submitted her paper on her new method to improve the purity of the drug "Wonder". Previously, she was able to show that the drug produced using her method had a contaminant level that was statistically significantly different to the government guideline figure of $\mu = 50$. However, one of the paper's reviewers has now said that she must compare her method with recent work by Professor B, who has also shown improvements in purity.

Professor A asks her researcher to produce 10 batches of the drug using Professor B's method, resulting in the following contaminant levels: (48.68 52.40 46.83 50.33 47.02 46.44 54.30 49.26 48.64 47.75), sample mean $\bar{x}_c = 49.164$, and sample standard deviation $s_c = 2.5414$. Professor A's method ($\bar{x}_t = 47.29$ and $s_t = 2.61$ for $n = 10$) seems to produce batches of the drug with fewer contaminants, but is the difference between her method and Professor B's method statistically significant?

To answer this question, we are going to carry out a Student's *t*-test to assess the difference between the means of two populations with unpaired samples. We use the subscript t to denote "test" batches produced using Professor A's method and the subscript c ("control") to denote Professor B's method. The test we are going to use assumes that both populations have the same variance. We have $s_t^2 = 6.82$ and $s_c^2 = 6.46$, so they are close.[3]

So, going through our checklist, we:

  ◼ *Examine the data*. The histograms are shown in Fig. 5.8.

---

[3] See Section 5.12 at the end of this chapter for a formal way of testing for equality of variance.

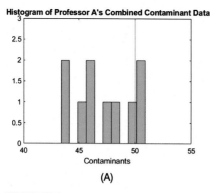
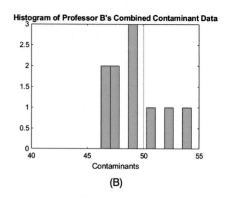

FIGURE 5.8
Histograms of ten batches of the drug "Wonder" produced using (A) Professor A's method and (B) Professor B's method.

■ *Formulate hypotheses and choose the degree of confidence.* Our null hypothesis is that there is no difference between the mean values of the populations from which the two samples were drawn, and the alternative hypothesis is that there is such a difference. We will work to 95% confidence.

■ *Calculate a test statistic from the data*: This has changed slightly ...

For the two-sample t-test, the equations to compute the test statistic are a little more complicated. Firstly, we have two standard deviations s_c and s_t, and we could have different sample sizes n_c and n_t. We need to calculate a pooled estimate of a combined standard deviation, which is a weighted sum of the individual standard deviations:

$$s = \sqrt{\frac{(n_t - 1)s_t^2 + (n_c - 1)s_c^2}{n_t + n_c - 2}}. \tag{5.3}$$

The test statistic is also altered slightly to account for our having n_c values from one sample and n_t from the other:

$$t = \frac{\bar{x}_t - \bar{x}_c}{s\sqrt{\frac{1}{n_t} + \frac{1}{n_c}}}. \tag{5.4}$$

So, for our data, we compute $s = 2.5769$ and $t = -1.6252$. Let us now return to our checklist:

■ *Compare the test statistic with a critical value and decide if we can reject the null hypothesis*: The number of degrees of freedom has changed slightly as we have had to calculate two mean values to obtain our t value. Therefore, we have $n_t + n_c - 2 = 18$ degrees of freedom. Looking at Table A.1, for $\alpha = 0.5$ and $df = 18$, we find that the critical value is 2.101. Because $|-1.6252| < 2.101$, we *cannot* reject the null hypothesis.

Therefore, unfortunately for Professor A, she is currently unable to show that her technique results in a statistically significantly different contaminant level from that of Professor B.

■ **Activity 5.6**

It is well established that smoking is associated with chronic obstructive pulmonary disease. Research has linked this process to a number of inflammatory signatures in exhaled breath condensate (EBC), one of which is nitrite concentration. Average nitrite EBC concentration was collected from eleven nonsmokers and nine smokers.

O5.D

Results for the nonsmokers were: $\bar{x}_{non} = 16208$ nmol/L, $s_{non} = 4862$ nmol/L. Results for the smokers were: $\bar{x}_{smoke} = 23176$ nmol/L, $s_{smoke} = 6763$ nmol/L.

Use a two-sample unpaired data t-test to determine whether there is a significant difference in the mean nitrite EBC concentrations between smokers and nonsmokers ($\alpha = 0.05$). ■

5.7.3   Paired vs. Unpaired t-test

So when should we use a paired or an unpaired data Student's t-test? Generally, paired t-tests are preferred as they have greater statistical power and make it easier to show statistical significance when the differences between samples are small compared to the variation within the samples. However, for practical reasons, it is not always possible to acquire paired data. For example, in Professor A's case, she had no way of pairing the two production processes, so she had to work with unpaired data. This is true in many real-world situations.

5.8   1-TAILED VS. 2-TAILED TESTS

All of the hypothesis test examples that we have seen so far have tested for *any* difference between the samples (or the sample and an expected value). We chose not to investigate which of the two was greater than the other. Sometimes we may be interested in this, and hypothesis tests can be applied in two different ways to reflect this need.

Hypothesis tests can be either *1-tailed* or *2-tailed*. Put simply, if we are interested in *any* difference between our two samples (or our one sample and an expected value), then we use a 2-tailed test. If we are interested in determining if a particular sample is either only *greater than* or only *less than* the other, then we use a 1-tailed test. Fig. 5.9 illustrates why these names are used. The curves represent a t-distribution for 10 degrees of freedom, and the shaded area in

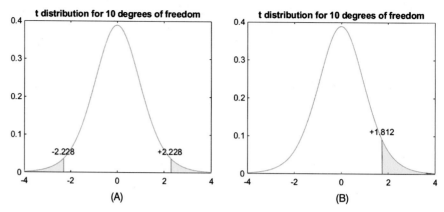

FIGURE 5.9
An illustration of 1-tailed and 2-tailed t-tests. The curve shown in both figures is a t-distribution for 10 degrees of freedom. (A) A 2-tailed test: the shaded area corresponds to the range of calculated t-values that would result in rejection of the null hypothesis. In this case, we are interested in finding *any* difference between our two samples. (B) A 1-tailed test, in which we are only interested in finding if a particular one of our samples is *greater than* the other. Note that the total shaded area is the same in both cases and corresponds to 5% of the total area (i.e. 95% confidence). However, for a 1-tailed t-test, a lower critical t-value results, making it easier to show significance.

both cases corresponds to 5% of the total area under the curve. The left-hand plot shows the 2-tailed case, and the right-hand plot shows the 1-tailed case. The critical t-value for 10 degrees of freedom and $\alpha = 0.05$ is shown as 2.228 for a 2-tailed t-test (we can look this value up in Table A.1). Therefore any computed t-value inside the shaded area will result in rejection of the null hypothesis. The right-hand plot shows how the critical t-value changes when we are only interested in one tail. We still need to have 5% of the total area outside of the critical t-value, so the critical value must be smaller in magnitude. For this reason, it is easier to show statistical significance when using a 1-tailed test than a 2-tailed test. The critical t-values given in Table A.1 are for 2-tailed t-tests. To use these same values for a 1-tailed test, we should double the significance level (e.g. if we want a significance level of 0.05, then we look up the critical value from the 0.1 column).

To illustrate the application of a 1-tailed test, we return to Professor A's original one-sample Student's t-test from Section 5.5. Recall that the absolute t-value was computed as 2.053, and we could *not* reject the null hypothesis because this was not greater than the (2-tailed) critical t-value of 2.776. Looking again at Table A.1, we find the 1-tailed critical t-value under the column for 0.1 significance level (this is double the actual significance level of 0.05). This is equal to 2.132, so in this case, it does not change the outcome of the test.

5.9 HYPOTHESIS TESTING WITH LARGER SAMPLE SIZES: THE z-TEST

The Student's t-test is widely used when the sample size is reasonably small (less than approximately 30). In these cases the sample distribution of the mean is known to follow a t-distribution. But what if our sample is large? In these cases the t-distribution tends toward a normal distribution. It is still possible to use a t-test for large sample sizes, and although Table A.1 does not go above a sample size of 36, critical t values for larger sample sizes can be found from a number of free online calculators.[4]

However, for large sample sizes, it may also be possible to use a z-test. The z-test is similar to the t-test except that it is only valid for large sample sizes and for cases in which the population variance is known. As it is not often that we know the population variance, the z-test is much less widely used than the t-test.

The procedure for applying a z-test is basically the same as that for a t-test, but the critical values are different. If we look at the table of critical values for the t-test (see Table A.1 in the Appendix), then we can observe that as the sample size increases, they *converge* (i.e. the differences between successive critical values get less). We can also see this convergence for 0.05 significance in Fig. 5.4. The values that the t-test critical values converge to are the critical values for the z-test, and these are provided in Table A.2. Note that these values are simply the number of standard errors that we need to go from the mean value in order that the proportion of the area under the normal distribution curve is equal to the degree of confidence. We already saw these numbers in Chapter 4 when we discussed computing confidence intervals for large samples (e.g. compare Fig. 4.8 with the values in Table A.2).

The assumptions of the z-test are similar to those of the t-test. First, the variable(s) being tested must be approximately normally distributed. However, as noted before, for the z-test, there is also an assumption that the population variance (i.e. the square of the standard deviation) is known. This means that the equations are slightly different. For example, the equation for the test statistic of the one sample z-test against an expected mean is

$$z = \frac{\bar{x} - \mu}{\sigma/\sqrt{n}},$$ (5.5)

which is the same as Eq. (5.1) for the t-test with the exception that we now use the population standard deviation σ rather than the sample standard deviation s.

---

[4]For example, see: https://mathcracker.com/t_critical_values.php.

Similarly, for the two-sample unpaired case, we have

$$z = \frac{\bar{x}_c - \bar{x}_t}{\sqrt{\frac{\sigma_c^2}{n_c} + \frac{\sigma_t^2}{n_t}}},$$

(5.6)

which is the same as Eq. (5.4) except that we now have two (known) population standard deviations (σ_c and σ_t) rather than one pooled estimate of the sample standard deviation.

For large sample sizes, the sample standard deviation can be a reasonable estimate of the population standard deviation, but in such cases a t-test will give similar results to the z-test. Therefore, it is fine to use a t-test for large sample sizes if we do not know our population variance. If we do know this, then a z-test may be preferable.

■ **Activity 5.7**

O5.E Researchers are investigating the link between genetics and cholesterol level. Their hypothesis is that a mutation in the LDLR gene is linked to high levels of cholesterol. Cholesterol levels (in mmol/L) have been measured from a group of 100 subjects who have the LDLR mutation. The cholesterol levels have been analyzed and found to be normally distributed. The mean cholesterol level of the group was found to be 5.31 mmol/L. From a previous study the population standard deviation of cholesterol levels is known to be 1.18 mmol/L.

Working to a 95% degree of confidence, use a z-test to determine whether it can be shown that the group of subjects with the LDLR mutation have a significantly different cholesterol level to the recommended safe level of 5 mmol/L. ■

5.10 SUMMARY

Hypothesis tests can be used to test for the statistical significance of differences between data. To do a hypothesis test, we must first form null and alternative hypotheses to be tested. We should also choose a degree of confidence (or significance level) to work to. Next, a test statistic is computed and compared to a critical value from a set of tables. To look up the critical value, we must define the number of degrees of freedom of the data. By comparing the computed and critical values of the test statistic the null hypothesis may be rejected or not.

Results of hypothesis tests can be wrong, and two types of error are possible. In a type I error, statistical significance is found when no such difference exists in reality. Type II errors occur when no statistical significance is found but there is such a difference in reality.

The most powerful type of hypothesis test is the parametric test, in which we assume that we know the underlying distribution of the data. The most common parametric test is the Student's t-test. This is based on the t-distribution, which is approximately the same as the normal distribution for large sample sizes but becomes less similar for small sample sizes. The t-distribution can be used to compute confidence intervals for small samples.

The test statistic for the Student's t-test varies depending on whether the test is using one sample, or paired or unpaired two-sample data. Paired t-tests are generally more powerful than unpaired t-tests for two-sample data.

Hypothesis tests can be 1-tailed or 2-tailed, depending on whether we are interested in any difference between two samples or just a difference in a particular direction. It is generally easier to show statistical significance for a 1-tailed test.

A z-test can be used instead of a t-test for larger sample sizes, but it assumes knowledge of the population variance. If the population variance is unknown, then a t-test should be used.

5.11 PARAMETRIC HYPOTHESIS TESTING USING MATLAB

There are built-in functions in the MATLAB Statistics and Machine Learning Toolbox for all of the tests and techniques that we have covered in this chapter. The sections below outline the basics of using these functions. Please see the MATLAB documentation for more details.

5.11.1 Student's t-test

There are two built-in MATLAB functions for performing t-tests: `ttest` is used for the one-sample and two-sample paired data cases, and `ttest2` is used for the two-sample unpaired data case.

One Sample:

```
[h,p] = ttest(x,m,'alpha',a,'tail',t)
```

Performs a one-sample t-test between the sample array `x` and the expected value `m`. The null hypothesis is that there is no difference between `m` and the mean of the population from which `x` was drawn. The alternative hypothesis is that there is such a difference. An `h` value of 1 is returned if the null hypothesis can be rejected, and 0 is returned if it cannot. The variable `p` contains the p-value, which represents the probability that the null hypothesis is true but the sample data occurred by chance. The extra optional pairs of arguments, `'alpha'`, a and `'tail'`, t, specify the significance level and number of tails of the test. The default value for the significance level is 0.05, representing 95% confidence. The default value for the type t is `'both'`, meaning a 2-tailed test.

If t is `'right'`, then it will perform a 1-tailed test for the mean of x being *greater than* m. It t is `'left'`, then it will perform a 1-tailed test for the mean of x being *less than* m.

Two-Sample Paired Data:

```
[h,p] = ttest(x,y,'alpha',a,'tail',t)
```

Performs a two-sample paired *t*-test between the samples x and y. The null hypothesis is that the means of the populations from which x and y were drawn are the same. The alternative hypothesis is that they are different. An h value of 1 is returned if the null hypothesis can be rejected and 0 otherwise. The extra optional argument pairs specifying a and t have similar meanings to those described before. A `'tail'` of `'left'` tests if x is *less than* y, whilst `'right'` tests if x is *greater than* y.

Two-Sample Unpaired Data:

```
[h,p] = ttest2(x,y,'alpha',a,'tail',t)
```

Performs a two-sample unpaired *t*-test between the samples x and y. The null hypothesis is that x and y come from normal distributions with the same mean. The alternative hypothesis is that their means are different. An h value of 1 is returned if the null hypothesis can be rejected and 0 otherwise. The extra optional argument pairs specifying a and t have the same meanings as described before.

5.11.2 *z*-test

```
[h,p] = ztest(x,m,s,'alpha',a,'tail',t)
```

Performs a one-sample *z*-test to determine if the sample x was drawn from a distribution with mean m and standard deviation s. The null hypothesis is that x does come from such a distribution. The alternative hypothesis is that it does not. An h value of 1 is returned if the null hypothesis can be rejected and 0 otherwise. The extra optional argument pairs specifying a and t have the same meanings as described before.

5.11.3 The *t*-distribution

The following built-in MATLAB functions can be used to perform calculations with the *t*-distribution.

```
y = tpdf(x,v)
```

Computes the value of the *t*-distribution with degrees of freedom v at points x.

```
p = tcdf(x,v)
```

Computes the value of the *cumulative distribution function* for the t-distribution at value(s) x. The cumulative distribution function represents the total area under the t-distribution from $-infinity$ to x. The argument v indicates the degrees of freedom of the t-distribution.

```
x = tinv(p,v)
```

Computes the value of the *inverse* cumulative distribution function of the t-distribution at value(s) p. The inverse cumulative distribution function takes a proportion p and returns the value x that has that proportion of the curve between it and $-infinity$. The argument v indicates the degrees of freedom of the t-distribution.

5.12 FURTHER RESOURCES

- One assumption made by the two-sample Student's t-test is that the variances of the two samples are equal. One way of testing this is using Levene's test for equality of variance. For further details, see https://en.wikipedia.org/wiki/Levene's_test
- If the assumption of equality of variance cannot be made, then Welch's t-test can be applied. For more information, see https://en.wikipedia.org/wiki/Welch's_t-test
- Free online calculators for critical z-test and t-test values are available at https://mathcracker.com/z_critical_values.php, https://mathcracker.com/t_critical_values.php
- The MATLAB documentation for the Statistics and Machine Learning Toolbox explains how MATLAB can be used to perform parametric hypothesis testing and contains a list of all implemented tests with explanations and examples that illustrate how to use them: http://mathworks.com/help/stats/hypothesis-tests-1.html

5.13 EXERCISES

Perform the following tasks, either by hand or using MATLAB, as specified.

■ Exercise 5.1

Verify Professor A's t-test for the "Wonder" drug's purity compared to the government guideline of $\mu = 50$ contaminant level. Use a significance level of $\alpha = 0.05$ and perform the one-sample t-test using MATLAB on: O5.D

1. The original 5-sample data; and
2. The 10-sample data.

■ **Exercise 5.2**

O5.D   Returning to the heart failure treatment research programme we introduced in Exercise 4.4 in Chapter 4, the researchers wish to test whether the LVESV values of the patients were significantly different from the clinical benchmark figure of 30 for healthy heart function. Use MATLAB to perform a one-sample t-test to test this hypothesis for both the pretreatment and posttreatment data ($\alpha = 0.05$). ■

■ **Exercise 5.3**

O5.D   Use MATLAB to perform a two-sample t-test to check for statistical significance of a decrease in the LVESV data between pretreatment and posttreatment ($\alpha = 0.05$). Should you use a paired or unpaired t-test? 1-tailed or 2-tailed? ■

■ **Exercise 5.4**

O5.D   In Activity 5.6, we introduced a study to investigate the link between exhaled breath condensate (EBC) and smoking. The original measurements were:

■ Nonsmokers: (19812 16015 15912 10546 23316 15220 11134 25655 14576 12016 14091)
■ Smokers: (22006 18467 12790 28499 26796 24924 14624 33167 27310)

Based on these data, use MATLAB to verify the calculation that you carried out by hand in Activity 5.6. ■

■ **Exercise 5.5**

O5.C   Working by hand, use the critical t-values from Table A.1 to compute the 95% confidence interval for the sample of 10 batches of the "Wonder" drug produced using Professor B's method: $\bar{x} = 49.164$, $s = 2.5414$. Next, do the same for Professor A's method. Comment on whether the confidence intervals indicate that the difference between the two methods was statistically significant. ■

■ **Exercise 5.6**

O5.C, O5.D   A group of researchers has developed a new "image-guided surgery" technology for neurosurgery. Image-guided surgery involves aligning preoperative images with the physical space of the operating theater and visualizing them to help surgeons perform operations more quickly and safely. The researchers would like to test if their technology results in shorter operation and recovery times, and to this end, they have gathered data from 21 patients. For each patient, the data consist of the operation time in minutes and the subsequent hospital stay in days. Seven of the patients underwent surgery using the new technology, and the other 14 had standard conventional surgery. The data can be found in the following files available from the book's web site:

- "standard_optime.txt": operation time for the 14 patients who underwent standard conventional surgery.
- "standard_recovery.txt": recovery time for the 14 patients who underwent standard conventional surgery.
- "image_guided_optime.txt": operation time for the 7 patients who underwent image-guided surgery.
- "image_guided_recovery.txt": recovery time for the 7 patients who underwent image-guided surgery.

Answer the following questions:

1. What type of data do we have here? (i.e. one-sample, two-sample, paired/unpaired?)
2. Read the four samples into MATLAB and plot histograms to visualize them. Do you think there will be a statistically significant difference in either the operation or recovery time?
3. Use MATLAB to compute 95% confidence intervals for the four samples. Now what can you say about the differences between them?
4. Use MATLAB to perform appropriate Student's t-tests to determine if either operation time or recovery time was significantly different for patients having surgery with the new technology.

Exercise 5.7

A research programme is using identical twin volunteers to try to establish a   *O5.D*
link between smoking and blood pressure. End systolic blood pressure data
have been gathered from 20 identical twins: for each pair of twins, one is
a regular smoker, and the other is a nonsmoker. These data are contained
in the files "pressure_non.txt" and "pressure_smoker.txt" available from the
book's web site.

1. First, assume that the data are *unpaired* and use MATLAB to perform a two-sample t-test to establish whether there is a statistically significant difference between the blood pressures of smokers and nonsmokers.
2. It could be argued that the fact that the volunteers are twins reduces the variability between them to the extent that the data can be considered to be *paired* data. Repeat the hypothesis test on the same data but this time use a paired t-test.

■ **Exercise 5.8**

O5.D

In this and the next exercise, we return to the study into the effect of vitamin B1 on Wernicke–Korsakoff syndrome patients introduced in Activity 5.4.

Assuming that the MMSE scores of the populations from which these samples were drawn have the same variance, state what type of hypothesis test you would perform to answer the following questions. For each, specify whether the data are paired/unpaired, one-sample/two-sample, whether the test should be 1-tailed/2-tailed, and the number of degrees of freedom.

1. Did the MMSE score of the test group decrease significantly after 6 months?
2. Was the MMSE score of the control group significantly different from that of the test group after 6 months?

■ **Exercise 5.9**

O5.D

Continuing with the Wernicke–Korsakoff syndrome example again, perform the first hypothesis test mentioned in Exercise 5.8 by hand, that is, determine if the MMSE score of the test group decreased significantly after 6 months (work to a 95% degree of confidence). Clearly state what your hypotheses are, show all working, and explain what the result of the test means.

(The mean and standard deviation of the difference between the before and after treatment MMSE scores for the test group were 3.15 and 0.94, respectively.)

■ **Exercise 5.10**

O5.E

Use MATLAB to repeat the one-sample z-test that you performed by hand in Activity 5.7. The original data are available in the file "ldlr_chol.mat".

■ **Exercise 5.11**

O5.B

We know that the t-distribution is a good approximation to the normal distribution for large sample sizes. In this exercise, we will verify this.

1. Use MATLAB to plot curves of the normal distribution (between, say, -5 and 5) and the t-distribution for different numbers of degrees of freedom (e.g. 3, 5, 10, and 30).
2. For each t-distribution, compute the standard deviation of the difference between it and the normal distribution.

FAMOUS STATISTICIAN: WILLIAM GOSSET

William Gosset is perhaps the most famous statistician of all time, but he is not usually referred to by his real name. He was born in Canterbury in the UK in 1876 and went on to study chemistry and mathematics at Oxford University. From 1899 onwards he worked for the Guinness brewery in Dublin, Ireland, applying his statistical knowledge to the selection of the best yielding varieties of barley.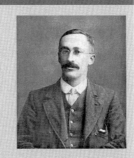

Gosset had a good relationship with Karl Pearson (see Chapter 1's Famous Statistician), and Pearson helped Gosset with a number of his papers, although he never fully appreciated their significance. Gosset's work generally dealt with very small sample sizes, whereas Pearson's work in biometrics generally had very large sample sizes. In fact, Gosset was for long the only figure on friendly terms with both Pearson and Ronald Fisher (see Chapter 8's Famous Statistician). However, despite his high standing in the field, Gosset's most significant work was not published under his own name. The reason for this is that another researcher at Guinness had previously published a paper that revealed some trade secrets of the company. To prevent further disclosure of confidential information, Guinness prohibited its employees from publishing any papers. After pleading with the brewery and explaining that his work was of no possible practical use to competing brewers, Gosset was allowed to publish, but only under a pseudonym ("Student"), to avoid difficulties with the rest of the staff. Thus, his most noteworthy achievement is now called Student's t-distribution, but otherwise it might have been named Gosset's t-distribution. The Student's t-distribution is the basis of the Student's t-test, probably most widely applied statistical hypothesis test in the world today.

> "I think that there are so very many things that we owe to 'Student' in the present statistical world. I would like to interest people in him, his practical mindedness and his simplicity of approach. It would be so easy for people to miss in the picture that large part he played simply by being in touch, by correspondence or personal meetings, with all the mathematical statisticians of his day."
>
> **Egon Pearson**

CHAPTER 6

Inferential Statistics III: Nonparametric Hypothesis Testing

6.1 INTRODUCTION

Up until now, all the hypothesis tests that we have seen in this book have been *parametric* tests. This means that (amongst other assumptions) they assume some knowledge of the distribution of the underlying population variable(s). Recall the distinction that we have made between the *population* and the *sample* of data that is drawn from it (refer back to Section 1.1 for a reminder). There are a range of hypothesis tests that do not require this assumption (or at least do not require such strong assumptions), and these are known as *nonparametric* tests. Nonparametric tests tend to be less powerful than their parametric equivalents. Therefore more data will typically be required to achieve statistical significance for the same degree of confidence. However, if we are not justified in making the necessary assumptions about the population distribution, then there is no alternative to using a nonparametric test, and in fact using a parametric test in such situations could cause misleading results.

Statistics for Biomedical Engineers and Scientists. https://doi.org/10.1016/B978-0-08-102939-8.00015-3

Table 6.1 Summary of the equivalence between common parametric and nonparametric hypothesis tests.

Parametric test		Nonparametric test	
Test	*Application*	*Test*	*Application*
One sample Student's t-test *(see Section 5.5)*	Mean of a population	Sign test *(see Section 6.2)* Wilcoxon signed rank test *(see Section 6.3)*	Median of a population
Two-sample paired Student's t-test *(see Section 5.7.1)*	Mean of a population of differences (paired data)	Sign test *(see Section 6.2)* Wilcoxon signed rank test *(see Section 6.3)*	Median of a population of differences (paired data)
Two-sample unpaired Student's t-test *(see Section 5.7.2)*	Mean of a population of differences (unpaired data)	Mann–Whitney U test *(see Section 6.4)*	Median of a population of differences (unpaired data)

The parametric hypothesis tests that we introduced in Chapter 5 were all based upon the *means* of the sample and population. The *median* (see Section 1.4) can be thought of as the nonparametric equivalent of the mean value for assessing the central tendency of a sample. When calculating a median, we disregard the actual values in the data and are only interested in their *rank* position within the data sample. In a similar way, nonparametric hypothesis tests often rank the data and compute a test statistic based upon the rank positions rather than the actual data values.

In this chapter, we discuss a number of the most commonly used nonparametric hypothesis tests (but readers should note that this is by no means an exhaustive list of such tests). Three of the tests that we will cover have approximate equivalences to the three parametric tests that we introduced in Chapter 5. These equivalences and the intended use of the tests are summarized in Table 6.1.

6.2 SIGN TEST

We will first consider the sign test. As can be seen from Table 6.1, this can be used in two different cases: for testing a single sample against an expected median value or for testing if the medians of two *paired* data samples are equal. Notice that the Wilcoxon signed rank test (see Section 6.3) can also be used in the same two cases. We will discuss later when we should choose which of these two tests, but for now, we will just note that the sign test is less powerful but more widely applicable than the Wilcoxon signed rank test. We will illustrate the use of the sign test for the one-sample case.

The basic idea of the one-sample sign test is straightforward and follows the checklist for hypothesis testing introduced in Section 5.2:

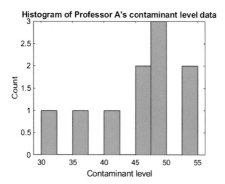

FIGURE 6.1
Histogram of contaminant levels in Professor A's "Wonder" drug: the data are now not normally distributed.

- *Form null and alternative hypotheses and choose a degree of confidence.* The null hypothesis is that the median of our population distribution is equal to a specified median value, and the alternative hypothesis is that it is different. The chosen degree of confidence determines the significance level, which will be used when deciding whether or not to reject the null hypothesis.
- *Compute a test statistic.* We count how many of the sample values are greater than or less than the specified median value. We then compute the probability of getting this number (or a more unlikely one) if the specified median was correct. This probability is our test statistic.
- *Compare the test statistic to a critical value.* For the sign test, our critical value is the chosen significance level. Therefore, if the probability is less than or equal to the significance level, then we reject the null hypothesis.

To illustrate this procedure, we return to the example of Professor A's "Wonder" drug introduced in Chapter 5. Recall that Professor A wanted to test if the contaminant levels in the drug were better than the government guideline of 50. Suppose that she has now produced a new batch of the drug and noticed that the new contaminant level data do *not* appear to be normally distributed. In this case, Professor A would need to use a nonparametric hypothesis test.

The contaminant level data resulting from Professor A's new production of the "Wonder" drug are as follows: (45.344 48.655 36.199 54.881 49.287 49.336 53.492 40.702 46.318 31.303). As always with hypothesis testing, our first step is to examine the data. A histogram of these new data can be seen in Fig. 6.1, and we can see that the data do *not* appear to be normally distributed and have a significant negative skew (see Section 1.5.3).

To perform the sign test, we first form our null and alternative hypotheses. We are interested in whether the sample median is *less than* 50, so our null hypothesis is that the sample median is not less than 50. The alternative hy-

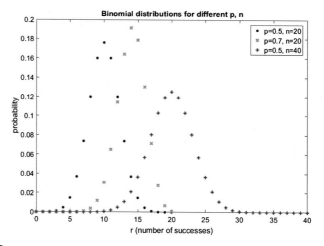

FIGURE 6.2

The binomial distribution for different numbers of trials (n) and probabilities of success (p).

pothesis is that it is. As we are interested in a difference in one direction only, we will perform a *1-tailed* test (see Section 5.8). We will work to a 95% degree of confidence, which means a significance level of 0.05.

Next, we compute our test statistic. To do this, we determine whether each sample value is greater than or less than the specified median of 50. Denoting values greater than 50 by "+" and those less than 50 by "−", we have: (− − − + − − + − − −). Counting these up, we have two pluses and eight minuses. If the null hypothesis were true (i.e. the median was not less than 50), what would be the probability that we would get this result (or a more unlikely one) by chance?

To answer this question, we must introduce the *binomial distribution*. In probability theory, the binomial distribution indicates the probability of the number of "successes" in n trials, each of which has a probability p of "success". The definition of "success" is arbitrary, but it is essential that each trial can have one of two possible outcomes, which are denoted as "success" and "failure". The binomial distribution specifies that the probability of r successes in n trials with a chance of success in a single trial of p is

$$P(r) = \frac{n!}{r!(n-r)!} p^r (1-p)^{n-r}. \tag{6.1}$$

Fig. 6.2 shows some examples of binomial distributions for different values of p and n.

For us, our "trial" consists of asking whether each sample value is greater than or less than the specified median value. We can define "success" as either "+" or "−" (the final result will be the same): we choose to define success as "−".

What we want to know is the probability of getting $r = 8$ *or more* "$-$" results in $n = 10$ trials. If our null hypothesis is true, then the chance of success in a single trial is $p = 0.5$. Therefore we compute:

$$P(8) + P(9) + P(10) = \frac{10!}{8!(10-8)!}0.5^8(1-0.5)^{10-8}$$
$$+ \frac{10!}{9!(10-9)!}0.5^9(1-0.5)^{10-9}$$
$$+ \frac{10!}{10!(10-10)!}0.5^{10}(1-0.5)^{10-10} = 0.0547.$$

This value 0.0547 is our test statistic. Essentially, this is telling us the probability of getting 8 or more values that are less than the specified median value of 50 if our null hypothesis were true.

The critical value for a 1-tailed sign test is simply the significance level 0.05. Comparing our test statistic with the critical value, we find that $0.0547 > 0.05$, so we *cannot* reject the null hypothesis. This means that Professor A has been unable to show that her contaminant levels are significantly better than the government guideline level.

Note that if we wanted to perform a 2-tailed test, then we would need to double the test statistic, since we want to compute the area under both tails of the distribution, that is, $P(0) + P(1) + P(2) + P(8) + P(9) + P(10)$ rather than just $P(8) + P(9) + P(10)$. Since the binomial distribution is symmetric, we can compute this by simply doubling $P(8) + P(9) + P(10)$. Therefore our test statistic would have been $0.0547 \times 2 = 0.1094$, and Professor A would still not have been able to show a statistically significant difference.

Note that this example was for the use of a sign test for testing a single sample against a specified median value. The same test can also be applied to two-sample paired data, by simply computing differences between the paired data values of the two samples and testing the hypothesis that the median of the population of such differences is zero.

■ Activity 6.1

Professor A asks her researcher to produce 10 more samples of the "Wonder" drug to attempt to show that her technique can produce the drug with lower contaminant levels than the government guideline. These data, combined with the existing data, resulted in 3 samples having a contaminant level of 50 or more (out of 20). Repeat the sign test on this combined sample: is the contaminant level now significantly lower than the guideline figure of 50?

O6.A

■

6.3 WILCOXON SIGNED-RANK TEST

Although the sign test can be used to test both one-sample and two-sample paired data, the Wilcoxon signed-rank test is more powerful than the sign test for these tasks because it makes use of the *magnitudes* of the differences rather than just their signs.

The Wilcoxon signed rank test was developed by Frank Wilcoxon[1] in 1945. We will illustrate its use using two-sample paired data. Following our checklist from Section 5.2, the basic idea behind the Wilcoxon signed-rank test is:

- *Form null and alternative hypotheses and choose a degree of confidence.* The null hypothesis is that the median of the population of differences between the paired data is zero. The alternative hypothesis is that it is not.
- *Compute the test statistic.* We do this by first computing the differences between the paired data samples; then we rank the differences *according to magnitude only*, that is, without regard to their sign; next, we sum the ranks of the positive and negative differences; finally, we pick the minimum of the sums as our test statistic.
- *Compare the test statistic to a critical value.* If the test statistic is less than the critical value, then we reject the null hypothesis.

Again, we will illustrate this procedure with an example. We will revisit the case we introduced in Section 5.7.1 for testing blood pressure data from patients suffering from hypertension. Two sets of data have been gathered: before treatment with a new drug and after treatment. The researchers now doubt that their data are normally distributed and so wish to try a nonparametric hypothesis test.

Our null hypothesis is that the median of the population of differences between the two sets of blood pressure data is zero. The alternative hypothesis is that it is not zero. Denoting the before treatment data as the control data and the after treatment data as the test data, our two samples are:

Control:	175.4	188.3	147.4	178.6	173.2	156.9	165.7	173.4
Test:	152.3	159.7	155.7	166.2	149.1	162.3	163.5	146.0

To compute our test statistic, we first compute the differences between the paired data, that is, test minus control. These are $(-23.1 \; -28.6 \; 8.3 \; -12.4 \; -24.1 \; 5.4 \; -2.2 \; -27.4)$.

Next, we rank these differences by magnitude and assign ranks to each difference value. This process is illustrated in Table 6.2. Note that the signs of the

---

[1] See the Famous Statistician at the end of this chapter.

Table 6.2 Wilcoxon signed-rank test: differences between two paired samples ranked by magnitude, with corresponding rankings.

Differences		−23.1	−28.6	8.3	−12.4	−24.1	5.4	−2.2	−27.4
Ranked differences		−2.2	5.4	8.3	−12.4	−23.1	−24.1	−27.4	−28.6
Ranks		1	2	3	4	5	6	7	8

difference values are ignored when ranking them, that is, they are ranked by magnitude only, but we remember the signs.

Next, we sum the rankings for the positive and negative differences (i.e. using the remembered signs). Referring to the ranks in Table 6.2, the sum of ranks for the positive differences is

$$T_+ = 2 + 3 = 5,$$

and the sum of ranks for the negative differences is

$$T_- = 1 + 4 + 5 + 6 + 7 + 8 = 31.$$

The minimum of these rank sums is T_+, which is 5, so this is our test statistic.

Now we look up a critical value in Table A.3 (see Appendix): for $n = 8$ and a significance level of 0.05 in a 2-tailed test, we have a critical value of 3. We compare our calculated and critical values: if the calculated value is less than the critical value, then we reject the null hypothesis. Since 5 is not less than 3, we cannot reject the null hypothesis in this case, so we cannot conclude that there is a significant difference between the two samples. Therefore, based on this test, we have not demonstrated that the new drug reduces blood pressure. Note the difference here with the parametric test on the same data (see Section 5.7.1): in that case, we were able to show statistical significance (on the assumption that the distributions were normal). Generally, significance is more likely to be shown with parametric tests than with nonparametric ones.

As we pointed out earlier, it is possible to use both the sign test or the Wilcoxon signed-rank test in either the one-sample case or the two-sample paired data case. To use the Wilcoxon signed-rank test in the one-sample case, we simply compute the differences by subtracting the expected median value being tested against from the sample. However, although both tests are applicable in both situations, the Wilcoxon signed-rank test is the preferred method as it makes use of the magnitudes of the differences rather than just the signs. It is important to remember that the Wilcoxon signed-rank test does make a stronger assumption about the data sample(s) being tested: it requires that the distribution of the differences is *symmetric*. If this can be shown to be not the case or if we have good reason to doubt that it is the case, then the sign test should be used.

■ The Intuition. Wilcoxon Signed-Rank Test

We have seen *how* the Wilcoxon signed-rank test can be used to test hypotheses about data that are not normally distributed, but *why* does it work like this?

The best way to understand the process underlying this nonparametric test is to think of it as converting the problem into one that can be addressed using a parametric approach. As noted before, the Wilcoxon signed-rank test makes the assumption that the distribution of differences between the two samples is symmetric. This assumption is important as it allows us to convert the original nonparametric problem into one that can be addressed by a parametric test. Note that the assumption is not saying that the distributions of the two samples are symmetric – we are only talking about the differences computed by subtracting the paired values (or the values from the expected median in the one-sample case).

Why do we need to make this assumption? An example of a distribution of differences is illustrated in Fig. 6.3A. If this is symmetric and the null hypothesis is true (i.e. the median of this distribution is zero), then there will be the same number of difference values above and below zero (this is the definition of a median). Therefore, the sums of the positive and negative ranks of these differences will be the same, that is, $T_+ = T_-$. What would be the expected value of these rank sums?

We can compute this using knowledge of the properties of an arithmetic series. The ranks for a sample of n numbers are simply the arithmetic series $1 + 2 + \cdots + n$. The sum of this series is $\frac{n(n+1)}{2}$, so we would expect the sums of either the positive or negative ranks to be $\frac{n(n+1)}{4}$ (i.e. half of the overall sum) if the null hypothesis were true. This value $\frac{n(n+1)}{4}$ is the mean of the distribution of rank sums. Importantly, *if the sample size n is large enough, then this distribution will be normal according to the central limit theorem*. The central limit theorem as we described it in Section 4.5 referred to the sample mean, but the same principle applies to the sum (which is just the mean multiplied by the sample size). Again, using knowledge of the properties of arithmetic series and some basic algebra, the standard error of the (normal) distribution of rank sums can be calculated as $\sqrt{\frac{n(n+1)(2n+1)}{24}}$. This is illustrated in Fig. 6.3B.

Now we have converted our nonparametric problem into a parametric one, and we can proceed in a similar way to our procedure for the Student's t-test (see Section 5.5). We compute our actual sum of ranks (i.e. from our data – for our blood pressure example, T_+ was 5) and compare this to the (now known) population distribution of rank sums. For our example, we have a population distribution of rank sums that has the following mean and standard error:

$$\mu = \frac{n(n+1)}{4} = \frac{8(8+1)}{4} = 18,$$

$$s.e. = \sqrt{\frac{n(n+1)(2n+1)}{24}} = \sqrt{\frac{8(8+1)(2 \times 8+1)}{24}} = 7.14.$$

Following the procedure outlined in Section 5.5, we compute our test statistic using Eq. (5.1):

$$t = \frac{\bar{x} - \mu}{s/\sqrt{n}} = \frac{5 - 18}{7.14} = -1.82.$$

This tells us that the rank sum we got from our data is 1.82 standard errors away from the expected rank sum. How likely is it that we would get this figure (or a more extreme one) if the null hypothesis were true?

For a one-sample Student's t-test with a sample size of 8 (i.e. 7 degrees of freedom), the critical value from Table A.1 for 0.05 significance is 2.365 (this is also shown in Fig. 6.3B). The magnitude of our test statistic (1.82) is not greater than the critical value (2.365), so we cannot reject the null hypothesis. This is the same result as we got using the simplified process outlined above. Note that the critical values in Table A.3 are simply precomputed values of the rank sums for the critical values of t-tests for different significance levels and sample sizes. ∎

■ Activity 6.2

A new drug has been developed that is intended to lower the cholesterol level of patients who have high cholesterol. Data have been gathered from 9 patients who had high cholesterol. The data consist of their cholesterol levels (in mmol/L) before and after taking the drug. The data are shown in the table.

O6.B

Cholesterol levels (mmol/L)								
Before 6.4	4.2	3.8	3.6	4.1	3.7	5.0	4.4	4.7
After 3.4	2.6	3.1	3.3	3.3	3.3	2.6	4.3	4.9

There is good reason to suspect that the data are not normally distributed. Perform a Wilcoxon signed-rank test to determine if there was a difference in cholesterol level as a result of taking the drug. Clearly state what your hypotheses are, show all working, and use a 95% degree of confidence in your test. ∎

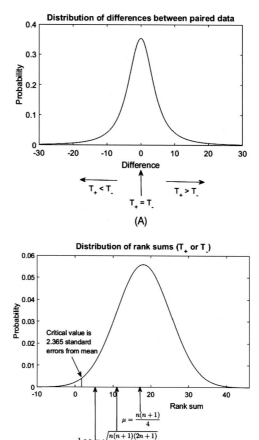

FIGURE 6.3
The intuition behind the Wilcoxon signed-rank test: (A) shows the (symmetric) distribution of differences between paired values from the two samples – the test statistics T_+ or T_- will be equal if the null hypothesis is true; (B) shows the distribution of rank sums, which is normal according to the central limit theorem – the computed test statistic is *not* beyond the critical value for the 0.05 significance level, so we cannot reject the null hypothesis.

6.4 MANN–WHITNEY U TEST

The next type of nonparametric test that we will consider is for two-sample unpaired data. The appropriate nonparametric test for this type of data is the Mann–Whitney U test. There are similarities between the Mann–Whitney U test and the Wilcoxon signed-rank test in that both involve ranking of values. However, since we are now dealing with unpaired data, it is not possible to

Table 6.3 Heights and weights of cohorts A and B. Cohort A suffered from malnutrition in childhood, and cohort B did not.

Height and weight data for cohorts A and B							
Cohort A: **Height (cm)**	180	170	163	171	167	155	174
Weight (kg)	78	76	80	78	66	73	74
Cohort B: **Height (cm)**	165	187	161	165	163	158	
Weight (kg)	83	82	100	83	74	101	

compute differences between values. Rather, we pool all original sample values and then rank them.

Following our checklist for hypothesis testing, we start off by forming our hypotheses:

- *Null hypothesis*: the two populations have identical distributions.
- *Alternative hypothesis*: the two populations have different medians, but otherwise are identical.

To compute our test statistic, we start off by pooling both samples (which are of sizes n_c and n_t for the control and test data, respectively) into a single large sample. We sort the data values in the large sample from $1, \ldots, n_c + n_t$ and then calculate the sums of the ranks from each individual sample. We use R_t to denote the sum of the ranks of the test sample and R_c the sum of the ranks of the control sample. Next, U_t and U_c are calculated using the following formulae:

$$U_t = n_t n_c + 0.5 n_t (n_t + 1) - R_t, \tag{6.2}$$

$$U_c = n_t n_c + 0.5 n_c (n_c + 1) - R_c. \tag{6.3}$$

The lower value of U_t or U_c is then compared with a critical value from a table. If the calculated value is *lower* than the critical value, then we reject the null hypothesis.

As a worked example, we consider a study investigating potential links between diet and physical development. Height and weight data have been gathered from two cohorts: one of subjects who had suffered from malnutrition in childhood (cohort A) and one of subjects who had not (cohort B). The height and weight data are shown in Table 6.3.

First of all, the research team wishes to determine if the *heights* of the subjects in cohorts A and B are different. Based on other findings of the study, the team has a good reason to doubt that all the populations from which these samples were drawn are normally distributed. Therefore, as we have unpaired data (i.e.

Table 6.4 Pooled ranks for the heights of cohorts A and B. Note what happens when ties occur.

Rank	1	2	3	4.5	6.5	6.5	8	9	10	11	12	13
Cohort A	155			163			167	170	171	174	180	
Cohort B		158	161	163	165	165						187

the subjects in cohorts A and B are different), we will use the Mann–Whitney U test.

To perform the test, we pool both samples and then rank the values from lowest to highest, remembering where each sample came from, as shown in Table 6.4. Note what happens when ties occur, that is, two data values are the same. In such cases the average rank is assigned to both values; for example, 4.5 is the average of the ranks 4 and 5.

We next sum up the ranks for cohorts A and B. Denoting cohort B as the control sample and cohort A as the test sample, we have:

$$R_c = 2 + 3 + 4.5 + 6.5 + 6.5 + 13 = 35.5,$$
$$R_t = 1 + 4.5 + 8 + 9 + 10 + 11 + 12 = 55.5.$$

We use these computed values $R_c = 35.5$ and $R_t = 55.5$, and the sample sizes $n_c = 6$ and $n_t = 7$ in Eqs. (6.2) and (6.3):

$$U_c = n_t n_c + 0.5 n_c (n_c + 1) - R_c = 27.5,$$
$$U_t = n_t n_c + 0.5 n_t (n_t + 1) - R_t = 14.5.$$

As a check that nothing has gone awry during the calculation, $U_c + U_d$ should equal $n_c \times n_t$. We have $U_c + U_t = 27.5 + 14.5 = 42$ and $n_c \times n_t = 6 \times 7 = 42$, so that is fine. We then take the lower of these two values, $U_t = 14.5$, as our test statistic.

The critical values for a 2-tailed Mann–Whitney U test at 0.05 significance can be found in Table A.4 in the Appendix. We find that our critical value is 6. As 14.5 is not less than 6, we *cannot* reject the null hypothesis, meaning that the team cannot conclude with 95% confidence that the heights of the two cohorts are different.

Note that Table A.4 is for a 2-tailed test at 0.05 significance level only. For other significance levels, a different table would be required. To use a 2-tailed table of critical U values for a 1-tailed test, we should double the significance level of the 1-tailed test, for example, we can use Table A.4 for a 1-tailed test at 0.025 significance level.

■ The Intuition. Mann–Whitney U Test

The intuition behind the Mann–Whitney U test is similar to that of the Wilcoxon signed-rank test described earlier: we transform the original non-parametric problem into one that can be addressed using a parametric approach. This time it is the U statistic (see Eqs. (6.2) and (6.3)), which is normally distributed and therefore can be assessed using a parametric test. The proof of this is beyond the scope of this book, but it was one of the key contributions of Henry Mann and Donald Whitney in their original paper on the test in 1947 [6]. The mean and standard deviation of the U distribution are

$$\mu = \frac{n_c \times n_t}{2},$$

$$\sigma = \sqrt{\frac{n_c n_t (n_c + n_t + 1)}{12}}.$$

From this we can proceed using a parametric test using these population distribution parameters and our computed U statistic (i.e. the minimum of U_c and U_t).

For instance, in our height example, we have $n_c = 6$ and $n_t = 7$. Therefore our mean and standard deviation can be calculated as

$$\mu = \frac{n_c \times n_t}{2} = \frac{6 \times 7}{2} = 21,$$

$$\sigma = \sqrt{\frac{n_c n_t (n_c + n_t + 1)}{12}} = \sqrt{\frac{6 \times 7 \times (6 + 7 + 1)}{12}} = 7.$$

So our population distribution for the U statistic for this example has a mean of 21 and a standard deviation of 7. Recall that our actual U statistic was 35.5. Again, we can ask how likely it is that we would have got this figure (or a more extreme one) if the null hypothesis were true? We answer this question by computing a Student's t-test statistic:

$$t = \frac{\bar{x} - \mu}{s/\sqrt{n}} = \frac{35.5 - 21}{7} = 2.07.$$

For a one-sample Student's t-test with 11 degrees of freedom (i.e. the sum of the two sample sizes minus two), the critical value from Table A.1 for 0.05 significance is 2.201. The magnitude of our test statistic is not greater than the critical value, so we cannot reject the null hypothesis. This is the same result as we got using the simplified procedure outlined before.

As before, it is important to remember that the critical values for the Mann–Whitney U test shown in Table A.4 are simply precomputed critical t-test values for the U statistic for different sample sizes. ∎

■ **Activity 6.3**

O6.C   Based on the data provided in Table 6.3, use the Mann–Whitney U test to determine if the *weights* of cohorts A and B are significantly different. Work to a 95% degree of confidence, clearly state your hypotheses, and show all of your working. ∎

6.5   CHI-SQUARE TEST

The nonparametric hypothesis tests that we have seen so far are suitable for ranked, discrete, and continuous data. Recall from Section 1.2 that some data are *categorical*, that is, their values are just labels with no ordering. What can we do if we wish to test hypotheses about categorical variables? The answer is that we can use a χ^2 (*chi-square*) test.

There are two cases to consider here: we may have one sample of a categorical variable and wish to test it against an expected distribution, or we may have two samples of (different) categorical variables and wish to test if their distributions are independent or not. We first deal with the one-sample case.

6.5.1   One-Sample Chi-Square Test

In the one-sample case, we have a single categorical variable. As a worked example, we use a clinical study that aims to investigate whether working in a high-stress job has an effect on people's blood pressures. A cohort of 500 subjects who work in high-stress jobs was recruited and had their blood pressures measured and categorized as *normotensive* (normal blood pressure), *hypertensive* (high blood pressure) and *prehypertensive* (slightly high blood pressure with an increased risk of developing hypertension). The variable in this case is the blood pressure category, and it can take one of three values, as described before. In the study, 255 subjects were found to be normotensive, 165 were prehypertensive, and 80 were hypertensive.

In a separate study of a random sample of the normal population the proportions of subjects who were normotensive, prehypertensive, and hypertensive were 63%, 25%, and 12%, respectively. We wish to know if those in high-stress jobs have blood pressures from the same distribution as the normal population.

The basic steps of this χ^2 test are similar to those for the other hypothesis tests that we have seen and are summarized as follows:

Table 6.5 Observed and expected values for blood pressure categories.

	Normotensive	Prehypertensive	Hypertensive
Observed frequencies, O	255	165	80
Expected frequencies, E	315	125	60

■ *Form null and alternative hypotheses and choose a degree of confidence.* For this x^2 test, the null hypothesis is that the sample data come from the expected distribution, and the alternative hypothesis is that they do not. We will work to a 95% degree of confidence.

■ *Compute the x^2 test statistic.* This is labeled *Calc x^2*, and an explanation of how it is calculated follows further.

■ *Compare our test statistic to a critical value.* We denote our critical value by *Tab x^2*, and we reject the null hypothesis if *Calc x^2* > *Tab x^2*.

For all x^2 tests, the test statistic *Calc x^2* is of the form

$$x^2 = \sum \frac{(O - E)^2}{E}, \tag{6.4}$$

where O is the *observed* frequency, and E is the *expected* frequency of values in each category. The sum (i.e. $\sum$) is performed over all possible values of the variable (in our example, there are three possible values).

The observed frequencies are simply the numbers of times we measured particular values in our study; for our example, we have 255 for normotensive, 165 for prehypertensive, and 80 for hypertensive. The expected frequencies are how many times we would expect to see each value *if the null hypothesis were true*, that is, the measured data fit the expected distribution. These can be calculated from the sample size and the expected proportions. For example, if the null hypothesis were true, then we would expect to see $500 \times 0.63 = 315$ normotensive subjects. Table 6.5 shows the observed and expected frequencies for our blood pressure example.

Now we calculate our x^2 test statistic using Eq. (6.4). We have:

$$x^2_{normotensive} = \frac{(255-315)^2}{315} = 11.43,$$

$$x^2_{prehypertensive} = \frac{(165-125)^2}{125} = 12.8,$$

$$x^2_{hypertensive} = \frac{(80-60)^2}{60} = 6.67,$$

$$\sum x^2 = 11.43 + 12.8 + 6.67 = 30.9.$$

Therefore our test statistic *Calc x^2* for this example is 30.9.

Table 6.6 Survival data for Ebola patients who did or did not take a new experimental drug.

	Survived	Died	Row totals
Took drug	20	7	27
No drug	14627	10365	24992
Column totals	14647	10372	25019

The critical values for a χ^2 test can be found in Table A.5 in the Appendix. The degrees of freedom for this type of test is $k - 1$, where k is the number of possible values of the categorical variable. We have $k = 3$ and therefore 2 degrees of freedom. From Table A.5 for 0.05 significance (i.e. 95% degree of confidence) we see that our critical value $Tab\ \chi^2$ is 5.991. We reject the null hypothesis if $Calc\ \chi^2$ is greater than $Tab\ \chi^2$. In this case, we clearly can reject the null hypothesis and conclude that the distribution of blood pressure categories is different for people in high-stress jobs.

6.5.2 Two-Sample Chi-Square Test for Independence

We now look at the second of the two cases mentioned earlier: we have two samples of (different) categorical variables, and we wish to test if they are independent. For this, the test is known as the χ^2 *test for independence*.

We will illustrate this test with a new example. In the Ebola virus epidemic in West Africa in 2014–15, an estimated 24,992 cases of Ebola were recorded. Of these, 10,365 cases resulted in the death of the infected person, and the other 14,627 resulted in survival. In addition to these cases, an experimental drug was used to treat 27 foreign health workers who became infected with the Ebola virus; of these, 7 died, and 20 survived. These data are summarized as a joint contingency table in Table 6.6. We wish to know if the survival rate for Ebola patients taking the new drug is significantly different to the survival rate for patients not taking the drug.

To answer this question, we form null and alternative hypotheses. Our null hypothesis is that the two categorical variables (i.e. *survived/died* and *took drug/no drug*) are *independent*, that is, there is no association between the variables. In other words, whether a person took the drug or not makes no difference to their survival chances. The alternative hypothesis is that they are not independent, that is, they are *associated*. In this example, we will work to a 0.05 significance level, that is, 95% confidence.

As for the one-sample case, the test statistic $Calc\ \chi^2$ is computed by comparing *observed* and *expected* frequencies. In this case, we perform this comparison for every cell in Table 6.6. The expected value E for each cell can be computed as

$$E = \frac{\text{Row total} \cdot \text{Column total}}{\text{Grand total}}. \tag{6.5}$$

Table 6.7 Expected values for survival data for Ebola patients who did or did not take a new experimental drug (assuming that the variables are independent).

	Survived	Died	Row totals
Took drug	15.807	11.193	27
No drug	14631	10361	24992
Column totals	14647	10372	25019

The expected values corresponding to Table 6.6 are shown in Table 6.7.

For each cell, we now compute a χ^2 statistic using Eq. (6.4). The value of *Calc* χ^2 is computed as the sum of all χ^2 statistics for all cells in the table. For our example this is

$$
\begin{aligned}
Calc\ \chi^2 &= \frac{(20 - 15.807)^2}{15.807} + \frac{(7 - 11.193)^2}{11.193} \\
&+ \frac{(14627 - 14631)^2}{14631} + \frac{(10365 - 10361)^2}{10361} = 2.6856.
\end{aligned}
$$

Finally, we compare *Calc* χ^2 with a critical value from Table A.5. For this type of χ^2 test, the number of degrees of freedom is equal to $(r-1)(c-1)$, where r and c are the numbers of rows and columns in our table, respectively (i.e. the number of different values each categorical variable can take). For our example, $r = 2$ and $c = 2$, so we have 1 degree of freedom. Consulting Table A.5, for a significance level of 0.05, our critical value *Tab* χ^2 is 3.841. Because *Calc* χ^2 (2.6856) is not bigger than *Tab* χ^2 (3.841), we cannot reject the null hypothesis. Therefore, there is no significant difference in survival rates between patients who took the new drug and those who did not.

■ The Intuition. The Chi-Square Test

Both types of χ^2 test that we have covered work on the same principle. They both compute sums of squared differences between expected and observed values. In mathematics, the distribution of a sum of the squares of a number of independent standard normal random variables is the χ^2 distribution, and an example of this is shown in Fig. 6.4. A large value of the χ^2 test statistic *Calc* χ^2 moves us to the right of this plot, and when we go beyond the critical χ^2 value (*Tab* χ^2), we conclude that such a value is unlikely to have occurred by chance and so reject the null hypothesis. The vertical line in Fig. 6.4 shows this critical value for a 95% degree of confidence, that is, the gray-shaded area represents 5% of the area under the curve. So we can see that a similar principle underlies the χ^2 test as underlies the *t*-test, but the distribution is different due to the way that the test statistic is calculated.

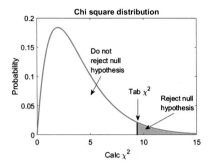

FIGURE 6.4

The χ^2 distribution and the critical χ^2 value $Tab\ \chi^2$. The null hypothesis is rejected when $Calc\ \chi^2$ is greater than $Tab\ \chi^2$. The vertical line shows the value of $Tab\ \chi^2$ for a 95% degree of confidence, i.e. the gray-shaded area represents 5% of the area under the curve.

Note also that χ^2 tests are always 1-tailed in that we only ever reject the null hypothesis for large values of $Calc\ \chi^2$: small values are consistent with the null hypothesis, and the values can never be negative. However, because we are dealing with *squared* errors, the test does not distinguish between the *direction* of the differences – it only determines if any difference exists. ■

■ **Activity 6.4**

O6.D   A new low-cost mobile ultrasound probe has been developed, and the development team wishes to determine if the image quality is the same as the existing probe. A sonographer has acquired 100 images with the new probe, and a radiologist has viewed them and classified them into three categories: *poor, acceptable*, and *good*. Of the 100 images, 7 were found to be *poor*, 16 were found to be *acceptable*, and 77 were found to be *good*.

Based on a previous study, it was found that, using the existing probe, the proportions of images in the *poor, acceptable*, and *good* categories were 5%, 17%, and 78%, respectively.

Use a one-sample χ^2 test to determine if images acquired using the new probe have the same distribution of image quality as those acquired using the existing probe. Work to a 95% degree of confidence, state your hypotheses, and show all working. ■

■ **Activity 6.5**

O6.D   A *pancreatectomy* is a risky surgical procedure to remove the pancreas. The operation is known to have a number of possible complications, and there is a significant postoperative mortality rate using traditional surgical techniques.

A new surgical technique has been developed with the aim of reducing the mortality rate. The new approach is based on the concept of image-guided surgery (IGS), which means to make use of preoperative images to guide the surgery. A number of patients who were considered to be high risk have undergone pancreatectomy using the new IGS technique. Mortality data have been gathered of the total number of patients who underwent traditional pancreatectomy in a single year, as well as the patients who underwent the IGS-based surgery in the same time period. These data are shown in the following table.

	Died	Survived
Traditional surgery	101	1108
IGS-based surgery	1	49

Use a χ^2 test for independence to determine if it can be concluded with 99% confidence that the type of surgery undergone influences the mortality rate. State your hypotheses and show all working.

6.6 SUMMARY

Parametric tests assume knowledge of the distribution of the underlying population. Nonparametric tests do not make such strong assumptions but tend to be less powerful than their parametric counterparts.

The sign test and the Wilcoxon signed-rank test can be used to either:

- Determine if a single sample has a median that is different from a specified value. (The parametric equivalent is the one-sample Student's t-test.)
- Determine if two samples of paired data have different median values. (The parametric equivalent is the two-sample paired data Student's t-test.)

The Wilcoxon signed-rank test is the preferred method, but it can only be used if the distribution of differences is symmetric.

The Mann–Whitney U test can be used to determine if two samples of unpaired data have different median values. A parametric equivalent is the two-sample unpaired data Student's t-test.

The χ^2 test can be used to test hypotheses about samples of categorical data. We have considered two cases: testing a single sample against an expected distribution and testing if two samples (representing different variables) are independent.

6.7 NONPARAMETRIC HYPOTHESIS TESTING USING MATLAB

There are built-in functions in the MATLAB Statistics and Machine Learning Toolbox for most of the tests that we have covered in this chapter. The sections below outline the basics of using these functions. See the MATLAB documentation for more detail.

6.7.1 Sign Test

The `signtest` function can be used to perform both one- and two-sample paired data sign tests.

One Sample:

```
[p,h] = signtest(x,m,'alpha',a,'tail',t)
```

Performs a sign test for a single sample x against a specified population median m using a critical value of a (default value 0.05). The null hypothesis is that there is no difference between the median of x and m. The alternative hypothesis is that there is such a difference. An h value of 1 is returned if the null hypothesis can be rejected. If the value of t is `'both'` (the default value), then the test will be 2-tailed. If t is `'right'`, then it will perform a 1-tailed test for the median of the sample being *greater than* m. If t is `'left'`, then it will perform a 1-tailed test for the sample median being *less than* m.

Two-Sample Paired Data:

```
[p,h] = signtest(x,y,'alpha',a,'tail',t)
```

As above, but it performs a two-sample paired data sign test, that is, it tests the medians of the populations from which x and y were drawn. If t is `'right'`, then it will perform a 1-tailed test for y being less than x. If t is `'left'`, then it will test for x being less than y.

6.7.2 Wilcoxon Signed-Rank Test

The `signrank` function can be used to perform both one- and two-sample paired data Wilcoxon signed-rank tests.

One Sample:

```
[p,h]= signrank(x,m,'alpha',a,'tail',t)
```

Performs a Wilcoxon signed-rank test for a single sample x against a specified median m. The null/alternative hypotheses and the meanings of all arguments are the same as for the corresponding use of the `signtest` function.

Two-Sample Paired Data:

```
[p,h]= signrank(x,y,'alpha',a,'tail',t)
```

As above, but it performs a paired data Wilcoxon signed-rank test between x and y. The null/alternative hypotheses and the meanings of all arguments are the same as for the corresponding use of the `signtest` function.

6.7.3 Mann–Whitney U Test

```
[p,h] = ranksum(x,y,'alpha',a,'tail',t)
```

Performs a 2-tailed Mann–Whitney U test between the data sets x and y. The null hypothesis is that x and y come from identical distributions. The alternative hypothesis is that their medians are different but the distributions are otherwise identical. An h value of 1 is returned if the null hypothesis can be rejected. The extra optional argument pairs specifying a and t have the same meanings as they do for the `signtest` and `signrank` functions.

6.7.4 Chi-Square Test

One Sample:

There is no built-in function to perform the one-sample χ^2 test in MATLAB. One way to perform the test is to compute *Calc* χ^2 using MATLAB commands and then to use the `chi2cdf` function to compute the area under the χ^2 distribution curve that is beyond the *Calc* χ^2 value. This can then be compared to the significance level to determine if the null hypothesis can be rejected. For example, the following code achieves this for the example that we went through in Section 6.5.1.

```
% Ultrasound image quality example
clear;

% sample size
n=500;

% expected values
ex_norm = n * 0.63;
ex_pre = n * 0.25;
ex_hyper = n * 0.12;

% observed values
obs_norm = 255;
obs_pre = 165;
obs_hyper = 80;

% chi^2 test
calc_chi2 = (obs_norm - ex_norm)^2/ex_norm + ...
            (obs_pre - ex_pre)^2/ex_pre + ...
            (obs_hyper - ex_hyper)^2/ex_hyper;
```

```
p = 1—chi2cdf(calc_chi2,2);
% (second argument is degrees of freedom)
% p=0.1.95e—07, which is < 0.05 so can reject null hypothesis
```

We compute a p value of 1.95e-07, which is smaller than the significance level of 0.05 for a 95% degree of confidence. Therefore we reject the null hypothesis, as we did when working by hand in Section 6.5.1.

Two-Sample Test for Independence:

```
[tbl,chi2,p] = crosstab(x1,x2)
```

Cross-tabulates two 1-D arrays representing categorical variables x1 and x2. The output tbl represents the contingency table (see Section 2.2.1), chi2 represents the χ^2 test statistic, and p represents the probability that any association between the two variables is due to chance. For example, for 95% confidence, the null hypothesis of independence can be rejected if p is less than 0.05.

For example, the following code listing performs the two-sample χ^2 test for independence on the Ebola case study that we introduced in Section 6.5.2.

```
% Ebola case study
clear; close all;

% first variable: drug = 1, no drug = 0
x1=[zeros(24992,1);ones(27,1)];

% second variable: survived = 1, died = 0
ebola_survival_control = [zeros(10365,1);ones(14627,1)];
ebola_survival_test = [zeros(7,1);ones(20,1)];
x2=[ebola_survival_control;ebola_survival_test];

% cross tabulation and chi square test
[tbl,chi2,p] = crosstab(x1,x2)

% p=0.1012 means high chance of deviation from expected
% results being due to chance, i.e. two variables cannot be
% said to be independent, so drug makes no difference to
% survival chance
```

6.8 FURTHER RESOURCES

- http://www.real-statistics.com/non-parametric-tests/: Although it uses Excel to illustrate the practical application of statistics, this web site contains some very good descriptions of the nonparametric tests that we have covered (and some others), including their mathematical foundations.
- The MATLAB documentation for the Statistics and Machine Learning Toolbox explains how MATLAB can be used to perform nonparametric hypothesis testing and contains a list of all implemented tests with

explanations and examples showing how to use them:
http://mathworks.com/help/stats/hypothesis-tests-1.html

6.9 EXERCISES

Perform the following tasks, either by hand or using MATLAB, as specified:

■ **Exercise 6.1**

The original data for Professor A's contaminant levels can be found in the file "profa_data.txt" available through the book's web site. Use MATLAB to:

O6.A

1. Visualize these data by plotting a histogram.
2. Verify Professor A's sign test that was performed in Section 6.2, that is, test if the median of the first sample of 10 contaminant level values is significantly less than 50.
3. The extra contaminant level data mentioned in Activity 6.1 can be found in the file "profa_extra_data.txt". Combine this sample with the first sample to make a new sample of 20 values. Use the combined sample to verify the sign test that you performed by hand in Activity 6.1, that is, is the contaminant level now significantly lower than the guideline figure of 50?

■ **Exercise 6.2**

A pharmaceutical company is developing a new drug to reduce the viral load in patients with HIV. In a pilot study, 10 subjects are treated with the drug, and after 4 weeks, their viral load was measured, yielding the following results: (297 120 101 120 278 133 275 302 287 323). Note that the results represent copies of the virus per ml. The aim of the study is to reduce this level to less than 305 units/ml.

O6.A

Assume that the data are not normally distributed and so a nonparametric test is required. For each of the following parts, first work out the answer by hand and then verify your result using MATLAB.

1. Perform a sign test on the data to demonstrate whether the study has been successful in lowering the viral load to below the 305 units/ml level.
2. The original viral load data for the same patients (i.e. before taking the drug) was (350 187 109 119 290 190 301 320 289 372). Perform a two-sample sign test to determine if the viral load was lower after taking the drug.

■ **Exercise 6.3**

O6.B   We return again to the heart failure treatment research programme we saw in Exercise 4.4 and Exercise 5.2. The researchers now doubt whether their LVESV data are indeed normally distributed and wish to verify their findings by performing a nonparametric hypothesis test. Use MATLAB to perform a Wilcoxon signed-rank test to determine, with 95% confidence, whether the pretreatment and posttreatment LVESV data come from distributions with different medians. Use the same data files ("lvesv_pre.txt" and "lvesv_post.txt") as before. Once you have done this, verify your result by repeating the test by hand.   ■

■ **Exercise 6.4**

O6.C   Use MATLAB to verify the Mann–Whitney U tests performed on the height and weight data in Section 6.4.   ■

■ **Exercise 6.5**

O6.C   *"Is Friday 13th bad for your health?"* [7]. The data in the table below are part of a study analyzing whether superstitions affect human behavior. The table contains data on the number of patients accepted into an Accident & Emergency department as a result of accidents on Fridays the 6th (control) and the 13th (test).

Month	Number of accidents	
	Friday 6th	*Friday 13th*
Jan	9	13
Feb	6	12
Mar	11	14
Apr	11	10
May	3	4
June	5	12

1. By hand, use a Mann–Whitney U test to determine whether the difference in median values between the number of patients admitted on the 6th and the 13th is statistically significant (95% confidence).
2. Use MATLAB to verify the result you obtained by hand.   ■

■ **Exercise 6.6**

O6.C   In Exercise 5.4, we introduced an example relating to EBC concentration in smokers and nonsmokers. The data for nonsmokers (in nmol/L) were (19812 16015 15912 10546 23316 15220 11134 25655 14576 12016 14091). Results for the smokers were (22006 18467 12790 28499 26796 24924

14624 33167 27310). These data can also be downloaded from the book's web site in the files "ebc_non.txt" and "ebc_smoke.txt".

Plot histograms of the two data sets using MATLAB: do they appear normally distributed? Try running a Mann–Whitney U test to determine whether the two data sets have different medians. ∎

Exercise 6.7

Use MATLAB to verify the result of the one-sample χ^2 test you performed by hand in Activity 6.4. ∎

O6.D

Exercise 6.8

A biomedical engineering company has developed a new robotic surgeon and wishes to determine if it can perform surgery as well as human surgeons. A trial has been performed on animals, in which 50 subjects had surgery by a human surgeon, and 50 by the robotic surgeon. Each surgery was classified as a *success* or a *failure*. The human surgeon had 46 successes and 4 failures, and the robotic surgeon had 42 successes and 8 failures. Perform a two-sample χ^2 test for independence to determine, with 95% confidence, if there is any difference in success rate between the robotic and human surgeons. First, perform the test by hand, and then verify your result using MATLAB. ∎

O6.D

Exercise 6.9

A research group has developed a new algorithm for automatic "segmentation" (i.e. delineation) of tumors from Computed Tomography (CT) images. The automatic segmentations enable the volumes of tumors to be calculated, which would be of interest to oncologists for the purposes of detecting and monitoring the progress of cancer. However, the volume calculations would need to be very accurate (an error of less than 5 mm^3) to be useful for clinical purposes. The research group has tested their new algorithm on a database of CT images, in which tumors have been manually segmented and accurate volumes calculated. This has enabled the production of a set of error values for the automatic tumor volume calculations. Now the research group would like to know if their technique has an error that is significantly better than the accuracy requirement of 5 mm^3.

O6.E

The error data are contained within the file "tumour_errors.txt", which is available from the book's web site. Choose an appropriate hypothesis test and apply it using MATLAB to answer the research group's question. ∎

Exercise 6.10

Positron emission tomography (PET) imaging enables in vivo quantitative measurements of radiotracer concentration and is commonly applied to monitor the progress of cancer. A common measure is the *standardized*

O6.D

uptake value (SUV): if the SUV of a tumor increases over time, then this means that the cancer is becoming more active. However, SUV values are strongly affected by the presence of motion artefacts in the PET images, so correcting for motion such as that caused by breathing is of interest. A research group has developed a new technique for breathing motion correction of PET images. PET images have been acquired from 15 patients, and SUV values calculated for their tumors. These data are contained in the file "suv_pre_correction.txt". The images were then motion corrected using the new algorithm, and the SUV values recalculated. These data are contained in the file "suv_post_correction.txt". Both data files are available from the book's web site. Using MATLAB, read in and visualize the data, and choose and apply an appropriate hypothesis test to determine if the new technique changes the SUV values. ■

■ **Exercise 6.11**

O6.D SUV values for clinical use are commonly computed by taking either the mean or maximum SUV value within a region of interest. Changes in SUV are computed by finding the difference in these values between two scans. Basing an assessment of tumor change on the mean or maximum SUV may be subject to noise in the images. A better way of testing if SUV values have changed may be using a statistical test based on all values within the region. A patient undergoing chemotherapy has had PET images acquired before and after treatment. SUV values for all voxels within a tumor region for the two images can be found in the files "suv_pre_chemo.txt" and "suv_post_chemo.txt" on the book's web site. Because the tumor may have changed size, the two files may contain different numbers of SUV values, and the values do not represent corresponding voxels. Doctors wish to know if the activity of the tumor has changed as a result of the treatment. First, use MATLAB to compute the mean and maximum SUV values to answer this question. Next, perform an appropriate statistical test to answer the same question. ■

FAMOUS STATISTICIAN: FRANK WILCOXON

Frank Wilcoxon was born in 1892 to American parents in Cork, Ireland. He had a difficult and unconventional early life. He grew up in New York and in 1908 ran away to sea, before jumping ship, then working as an oil well worker and subsequently as a tree surgeon. In 1917 he moved to Pennsylvania to study at a military college before leaving to work for an explosives company during World War I. Finally, in 1920 he enrolled at Rutgers University to study chemistry. He graduated and went on to gain a PhD in physical chemistry from Cornell University in 1924 at the age of 32.

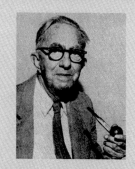

Credit: Famous Statistician: Frank Wilcoxon, From https://en.wikipedia.org/wiki/Frank_Wilcoxon#/media/File:FrankWilcoxon.png, Image taken from Karas, J. & Savage, I.R. (1967) Publications of Frank Wilcoxon (1892–1965). Biometrics 23(1): 1–10

His first job after completing his PhD was at the Boyce Thompson Institute for Plant Research, where he was assigned to investigate the use of copper compounds as fungicides. Here he worked alongside William Youden (see Chapter 3's Famous Statistician), and they both studied the statistical work of Ronald Fisher (see Chapter 8's Famous Statistician). Wilcoxon gradually became more interested in statistics, culminating in 1945 with the publication of his most well-known statistical paper. This described the now famous Wilcoxon signed-rank test, and even the initial version of the Mann–Whitney U test. This work was later extended to arbitrary sample sizes by Henry Mann and his student Donald Ransom Whitney. For this reason, the Mann–Whitney U test is also sometimes called the Mann–Whitney–Wilcoxon (MWW) test or the Wilcoxon rank-sum test. Frank Wilcoxon died in 1965 after a brief illness.

CHAPTER 7

Inferential Statistics IV: Choosing a Hypothesis Test

LEARNING OBJECTIVES

At the end of this chapter, you should be able to:

O7.A Interpret a quantile–quantile plot of sample data against a theoretical distribution and produce one using MATLAB

O7.B Compute the probability plot correlation coefficient between two distributions using MATLAB

O7.C Compute skew values by hand and using MATLAB, and interpret them to decide how close sample data are to a normal distribution

O7.D Compute z-values of a sample by hand and using MATLAB, and use them to decide how close the sample is to a normal distribution

O7.E Apply the Shapiro–Wilk test to sample data by hand and using MATLAB, to test if the sample fits a normal distribution

O7.F Apply the chi-square test to sample data by hand and using MATLAB, to test if the sample fits a normal distribution

O7.G Make appropriate use of tools to decide which hypothesis test to use

7.1 INTRODUCTION

We have now covered most of the main concepts of parametric and nonparametric hypothesis testing. We know that it is important to choose an appropriate test to ensure that we gain the maximum statistical power but that we do not violate any assumptions of the test we choose. So far we have just used simple "intuitive" ways of assessing our data to decide which type of test to use. For instance, we have plotted histograms of the sample data and visually inspected their distribution. However, sometimes this approach gives unclear results, and we would like to be more precise in our assessment. In this chapter, we look at more powerful tools that we can use to help us choose the best hypothesis test. As it is the most common criterion for choosing hypothesis tests, we focus on tools that can help us to decide whether our data fit a normal distribution. In particular, we would like to demonstrate that the population variable of inter-

147

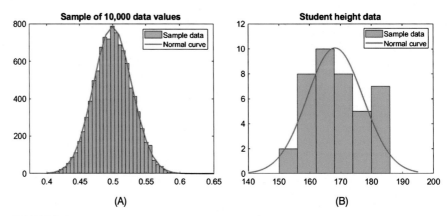

FIGURE 7.1
(A) Histogram of a sample of 10,000 data values with $\bar{x} = 0.5$ and $s = 0.029$. The curve shows the probability distribution function from a normal distribution with $\mu = 0.5$ and $\sigma = 0.029$. (B) Histogram of the student height data with sample size 40 and $\bar{x} = 168.25$, $s = 9.1083$. The curve shows a normal probability distribution function with $\mu = 168.25$ and $\sigma = 9.1083$. Note that both distribution curves have been scaled along the y-axis, so that they can be directly compared with the histograms.

est is normally distributed, as this is a key assumption of the Student's t-test. However, since we typically do not have full access to the population data, we can only assess our sample data, and we make the assumption that its distribution approximates the population distribution, which is reasonable since it is a random representative sample of the population.

7.2 VISUAL METHODS TO INVESTIGATE WHETHER A SAMPLE FITS A NORMAL DISTRIBUTION

7.2.1 Histograms

We have already seen the use of histograms to assess sample distributions several times in this book, so they are one obvious way to assess if data fit a normal distribution. Figs. 7.1A and 7.1B show histograms of sample data together with normal probability distribution functions with mean and standard deviation equal to the sample mean and standard deviation. Fig. 7.1A shows a sample with 10,000 data values. The sample distribution seems to fit well to a normal distribution. In this case, we might feel confident in applying parametric hypothesis tests to answer questions about the data. However, Fig. 7.1B shows the student height data that we first saw in Chapter 1. Would we be justified in assuming that this sample comes from a normal distribution? We will now consider further ways to help us to answer such questions.

7.2.2 Quantile–Quantile Plots

Histograms such as those shown in Fig. 7.1 are one visual way to assess similarity to a normal distribution. An alternative way is the *quantile–quantile plot*. We came across quartiles in Chapter 1 when discussing measures of variation for skewed data. We calculated the upper and lower quartiles and the median. These were defined as the data values which had:

- $\frac{1}{4}$ of the data values below it: *lower quartile*
- $\frac{2}{4}$ of the data values below it: *median*
- $\frac{3}{4}$ of the data values below it: *upper quartile*

The concept of a *quantile* is related to that of a *quartile*. A *quantile* is the generic name for a value which has $\frac{k}{q}$th of the data values below it (where q is the number of quantiles calculated, and $k = 1, \ldots, q - 1$). For example, we can compute the 95% quantile, which is the data value at which $\frac{95}{100}$ of the data values lie below that value (i.e. $q = 100$ and $k = 95$). The lower quartile, median, and upper quartile correspond to the 25%, 50%, and 75% quantiles, respectively.

For example, consider Fig. 7.2. Fig. 7.2A shows a uniform distribution between -5 and $+5$ (in blue). The black vertical lines indicate the values of the quantiles for $10\%, 20\%, \ldots, 90\%$ or, in other words, the values that have $\frac{10}{100}$, $\frac{20}{100}, \ldots, \frac{90}{100}$ of the distribution below them. Fig. 7.2B shows a standard normal distribution (i.e. a normal distribution with $\mu = 0$ and $\sigma = 1$) with the same quantiles. Notice how the quantiles for the uniform distribution are evenly spaced because the height of the distribution does not change, whereas those for the normal distribution are more closely spaced near the center of the distribution where the curve is higher. *The area under the curve between successive quantiles is the same in both figures*, that is, 10% of the total area.

We can produce a quantile–quantile plot (often called a *Q–Q plot*) by calculating the quantile values from two samples, or a sample and a theoretical distribution (e.g. normal distribution), and plotting the corresponding quantile values against each other. If the two samples come from the same distribution, then the plot should approximately show a straight line along $y = x$. Fig. 7.3 shows Q–Q plots for the two distributions shown in Fig. 7.1, both against a standard normal distribution.

How should we interpret these Q–Q plots? As noted before, if the two distributions are the same, then the Q–Q plot will show a straight line through the origin at 45°. The closer we are to this case, the closer the distributions are. However, in addition to this, certain shapes in the Q–Q plot imply particular types of difference between the distributions:

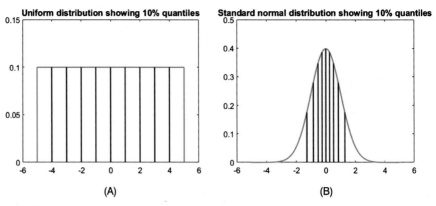

FIGURE 7.2
(A) A uniform distribution between -5 and $+5$ with quantiles shown at 10% intervals, that is, 10%, 20%, etc. (B) A standard normal distribution (i.e. $\mu = 0$, $\sigma = 1$) showing the same quantile values.

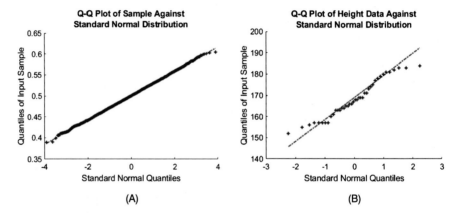

FIGURE 7.3
Q–Q plots for sample data against a standard normal distribution. (A) Sample data from Fig. 7.1A; (B) student height data from Fig. 7.1B.

- A straight line that is not at 45° and/or does not go through the origin implies that the distributions would be the same if a linear transformation was applied to one sample. If we are comparing a sample to a normal distribution, then this means that we have chosen the wrong mean and standard deviation for the normal distribution: if we chose the correct mean and standard deviation, then the Q–Q plot would show an ideal match.

- An arc shape in the Q–Q plot is the result of one distribution having a higher skew (see Section 1.5.3) than the other. This is illustrated by the example of a Q–Q plot between samples from normal and gamma distributions shown in Fig. 7.4.

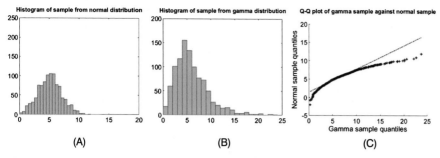

FIGURE 7.4

(A) A sample from a normal distribution with $\mu = 5$ and $\sigma = 2$; (B) a sample from a gamma distribution with shape parameter 3 and scale parameter 2; and (C) a Q–Q plot of the gamma sample against the normal sample. Notice how the higher skew of the gamma distribution causes an arc shape in the Q–Q plot.

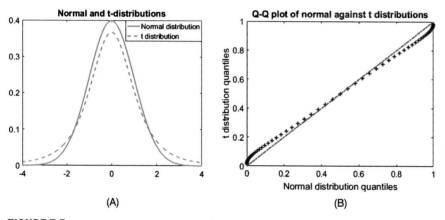

FIGURE 7.5

(A) Probability distribution functions for the normal distribution and a t-distribution with 3 degrees of freedom; (B) Q–Q plot for the same two distributions. Notice how the longer tails of the t-distribution cause an "S" shape in the Q–Q plot.

■ An "S" shape in the Q–Q plot indicates that one distribution has longer tails than the other. For example, Fig. 7.5 shows a Q–Q plot of samples from a normal distribution and a t-distribution with 3 degrees of freedom (see Section 5.4). The curves at the ends of the Q–Q plot make an "S" shape, which is caused by the different quantile values at the outer ends of the distribution.

We will now introduce a case study for this chapter and use it to illustrate the Q–Q plot. We return to Professor A and her attempts to revolutionize the

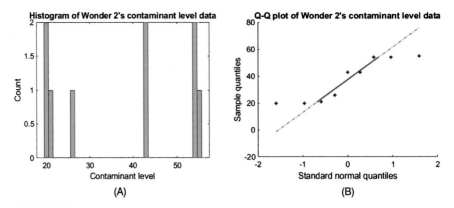

FIGURE 7.6
Analysis of Professor A's new "Wonder 2" contaminant level data: (A) histogram and (B) Q–Q plot. The Q–Q plot is against theoretical values from a standard normal distribution.

world of drug production. She has now given her researcher more freedom and asked him to come up with his own drug production technique. The result is a new drug, known as "Wonder 2". Nine batches of "Wonder 2" have been produced, and the contaminant level data are as follows: (21 54 20 55 20 54 26 43 43).

Fig. 7.6 shows a histogram and a Q–Q plot of these sample data against a standard normal distribution. As before, the Q–Q plot shows a cross for each quantile value, but note that this plot only shows 9 different quantile values. This is because there are only 9 values in the sample; therefore each data value is itself a quantile. For example, the 3rd smallest value has two values below it, 6 values above it, and 1 value equal to it (i.e. itself). So we can view this as the $\frac{2.5}{9}$th quantile, and we can find the corresponding quantile value from the standard normal distribution to plot it against. Similarly, the other data values represent the $\frac{0.5}{9}$th, $\frac{1.5}{9}$th, etc. quantiles.

Recall that any straight line in the Q–Q plot will indicate that the data come from a normal distribution (possibly with different mean and standard deviation). However, for these data, this does not seem to be the case, as is confirmed by the histogram which shows three distinct peaks.

Although Q–Q plots allow us to make a more informed assessment of whether data fit a normal distribution, there is still a significant element of subjectivity in this assessment, and this will be the case for any visual method. In the next section, we will introduce methods that can *quantify* how well the data fit the distribution, and even test hypotheses about the goodness-of-fit to the distribution.

■ **Activity 7.1**

Four samples have been drawn from unknown population distributions. The images below show their histograms and Q–Q plots. Match each histogram to its corresponding Q–Q plot.

O7.A

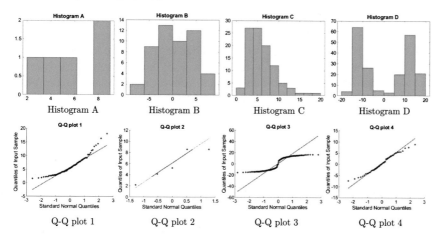

Q-Q plot 1   Q-Q plot 2   Q-Q plot 3   Q-Q plot 4

7.3 NUMERICAL METHODS TO INVESTIGATE WHETHER A SAMPLE FITS A NORMAL DISTRIBUTION

Numerical techniques have clear advantages over the visual methods that we have seen in the previous section. By quantifying (i.e. putting numbers to) how well data fit a particular distribution comparisons can be made between different samples in terms of how well they fit the distribution, and we can even think about ways of testing particular hypotheses about the fit.

In this section, we consider a number of numerical techniques that can be used to quantify some aspects of the sample distribution to help us to make more informed decisions about how close they are to a normal distribution.

7.3.1 Probability Plot Correlation Coefficient

The first numerical technique is actually derived from the Q–Q plot. The *probability plot correlation coefficient* (PPCC) is the Pearson's correlation coefficient of the data plotted in the Q–Q plot. We introduced the Pearson's correlation coefficient (or Pearson's r) in Section 2.4.1 as a measure of linear dependence between two variables. Recall that the Pearson's r value will be equal to 1 (or -1) whenever there is a linear relationship between two sets of data. For our Q–Q plot, any straight line means that our two distributions fit perfectly (or would do if an appropriate linear transform were applied to one of the data sets). Therefore, the Pearson's r value of the quantile data should be a good measure of how well the distributions match.

Let us return to our Professor A case study to illustrate this. For the sample data, the quantiles are the data values themselves: (20 20 21 26 43 43 54 54 55).

How can we compute the corresponding quantiles for the standard normal distribution? What we want to know is what values of the standard normal distribution have the same proportions of values below them as the quantile values for our sample. As explained in the previous section, for a sample of size n, the proportions are $\frac{0.5}{n}, \frac{1.5}{n}, \ldots, \frac{n-0.5}{n}$. Based on these proportions and the equation for a normal distribution, we can determine that the standard normal distribution quantiles are $(-1.593 \ -0.967 \ -0.59 \ -0.282 \ 0 \ 0.282 \ 0.59 \ 0.967 \ 1.593)$.

Calculating the Pearson's r value between these two sets of quantile values results in a PPCC of 0.9205. But what does this mean? What is an acceptable value for PPCC? In truth, there is no clear answer to this question, but a very high value (e.g. 0.99) would suggest that the sample distribution and the test distribution *were* similar. On the other hand, a much lower value (e.g. 0.75) would definitely suggest that they were *not*. Our value of 0.9205 is probably inconclusive, so it would be useful to perform some further analysis before making a final decision about the distribution of our sample.

7.3.2 Skew Values

Computing the *skew* of a sample is a quick test that we can use to test how *symmetric* its distribution is. We already saw one way to calculate skew in Section 1.5.3, which we reproduce here for convenience:

$$\text{skew} = \frac{3(\bar{x} - \text{median})}{s}.$$

If the skew is not between -1 and 1, then the distribution is not very symmetric and so may well not be normal.

Let us compute the skew of Professor A's latest contaminant level data. We have $\bar{x} = 37.33$, median $= 43$, $s = 15.52$, and therefore skew $= \frac{3(37.33-43)}{15.52} = -1.0951$. From this it seems as if our distribution has a significant negative skew, so it is still not looking good for it to fit to a normal distribution.

7.3.3 z-values

A further numerical test can be carried out by converting our sample data into z-values, as defined by the equation

$$z_i = \frac{x_i - \bar{x}}{s}. \tag{7.1}$$

This equation transforms our sample so that it has a mean of 0 and a standard deviation of 1. Therefore the z-values indicate how many standard deviations each value is away from the mean of the sample.[1] If our data are actually from a normal distribution, then from the properties of this distribution (see Fig. 4.5B) we know the percentages of values that should be less than 1, 2, 3, and 4 standard deviations from the mean, which are 68.3%, 95.4%, 99.7%, and 99.994%, respectively.

A quick check to see if our data come from a normal distribution is to look at the maximum magnitude of the z-values (i.e. ignoring their signs). It is very unlikely that we would obtain many z-values with magnitude 3 or more from a normal distribution unless we have a very large sample (we would only expect 3 data points with a z-value magnitude above 3 in a sample of 1,000, and we would need samples of 10,000 before we would expect to obtain a z-value magnitude above 4). Therefore large z-scores from small samples are an indication that our data may not be from a normal distribution.

Let us return to our case study. Our original data were

(21 54 20 55 20 54 26 43 43)

We transform these data to z-values using Eq. (7.1), resulting in

(−1.052 1.074 −1.117 1.138 −1.117 1.074 −0.73 0.365 0.365)

We can see straight away that we do not have any very large z-values. This seems promising at first. However, for our sample size of 9, we would expect to see $(1 − 0.68) \times 9 = 2.88$ values beyond 1 standard deviation. We have 6 values that are more than 1 standard deviation from the mean. This suggests that the distribution from which our sample was taken may have longer tails than a normal distribution.

■ Activity 7.2

A company has developed a new surgical technique for inserting hip implants. The angular error of the placement can be assessed postoperatively using x-ray imaging. Error data (in degrees) have been gathered from 9 patients who underwent the new surgery. The data are shown in the table below.   *O7.C, O7.D*

Angular error (degrees)								Mean	Std. dev.	Median
8	3	2	2	4	1	1	2	2.88	2.3	2

---

[1] Note the similarity of Eq. (7.1) with Eq. (5.5) in Section 5.9. Whereas the statistic in the z-test computes the number of *standard errors* our mean is from the expected mean, z-values compute how many *standard deviations* each sample value is from the sample mean.

1. Compute a skew value for the alignment error data. Comment on the result.
2. Compute z-values for the same data. Again, comment on the results with regard to whether the data are likely to be normally distributed. ◼

7.3.4 Shapiro–Wilk Test

All of the above techniques can provide useful information to help us to decide whether or not sample data were likely to have come from a normal distribution. However, sometimes the answer is still unclear, and it would be useful to have a way to make a formal decision as to whether this is likely to be the case or not. There are a number of more sophisticated methods to help us to answer such questions. A commonly used one for small samples is the *Shapiro–Wilk test*.

The Shapiro–Wilk test is a hypothesis test, and so we will follow the checklist for hypothesis testing that we first introduced in Section 5.2.

- *Form null and alternative hypotheses and choose a degree of confidence*: For the Shapiro–Wilk test, the null hypothesis is that the sample comes from a normal distribution, and the alternative hypothesis is that it does not. We can choose any degree of confidence, but common choices are 95% and 99%.
- *Compute a test statistic*: We do this by first ranking the sample values in increasing order – we denote these ranked data by $(x_{(1)} \ x_{(2)} \ \ldots \ x_{(n-1)} \ x_{(n)})$, where n is the sample size. Next, we calculate $b = a_1(x_{(n)} - x_{(1)}) + a_2(x_{(n-1)} - x_{(2)})\ldots$, where $a_1, a_2, \ldots$ are the coefficients from Table A.6 (see Appendix). Finally, the test statistic is computed as Calc $W = \frac{b^2}{(n-1)s^2}$, where s is the sample standard deviation.
- *Compare the test statistic with a critical value*: The critical W values for a Shapiro–Wilk test are shown in Table A.7 in the Appendix. We denote the critical value by Tab W.
- If Calc W > Tab W, then we do *not* reject the null hypothesis.

We will illustrate this process using the contaminant level data for Professor A's new drug "Wonder 2". We will work to a 95% degree of confidence, or 0.05 significance. The test statistic is calculated by following the steps outlined above:

- Rank the data: (20 20 21 26 43 43 54 54 55).
- Using coefficients from Table A.6 for $n = 9$, we calculate $b = 0.5888(55 - 20) + 0.3244(54 - 20) + 0.1976(54 - 21) + 0.0947(43 - 26) = 39.7683$.
- Calculate the test statistic: Calc $W = \frac{39.7683^2}{(9-1)15.52^2} = 0.8203$.

- Look up the critical W value in Table A.7: for $n = 9$, 0.05 significance, Tab $W = 0.829$.
- Because Calc $W <$ Tab W (i.e. $0.8203 < 0.829$), we *reject the null hypothesis*, that is, we conclude with 95% confidence that our data are *not* from a normal distribution.

This conclusion confirms our earlier suspicions based on the Q–Q plot, PPCC, skew, and z-values.

■ The Intuition. Shapiro–Wilk Test

The Shapiro–Wilk test is essentially a *goodness-of-fit* test. That is, it examines how close the sample data fit to a normal distribution. It does this by ordering and *standardizing* the sample (*standardizing* refers to converting the data to a distribution with mean $\mu = 0$ and standard deviation $\sigma = 1$). If the sample data perfectly fit a normal distribution, then after this ordering and standardization process the sample values would be regularly spaced quantile values of the standard normal distribution (see Section 7.2.2, in particular, the explanation of how to compute quantiles for Professor A's contaminant level data). The Shapiro–Wilk test statistic (Calc W) is basically a measure of how well the ordered and standardized sample quantiles fit the standard normal quantiles. The statistic will take a value between 0 and 1 with 1 being a perfect match. This is why a small value of Calc W will result in rejection of the null hypothesis of normality. The equation for Calc W given above, which is based on the coefficients in Table A.6, basically performs the standardization and calculation of the goodness-of-fit. Therefore, there is a close link between the Shapiro–Wilk test and Q–Q plots, which offer a visual assessment of this goodness-of-fit using quantiles.   ■

Note that the result of the Shapiro–Wilk test should not be taken as being 100% reliable (no hypothesis test should). There will be cases where the test will give a misleading result. Therefore the Shapiro–Wilk test should never be used on its own – it should always be interpreted along with the results of graphical and numerical tools. In many cases, it will be obvious from the graphical and numerical tools that the data are (or are not) normally distributed, so the Shapiro–Wilk test will be unnecessary. It can be useful, however, when the results of the graphical and numerical tools are inconclusive.

■ Activity 7.3

In Activity 7.2, we introduced the error data for a new surgical technique for inserting hip implants. For convenience, the data are shown again in the following table.

O7.E

Angular error (degrees)								Mean	Std. dev.	Median
8	3	2	2	4	1	1	2	2.88	2.3	2

Perform a Shapiro–Wilk test to determine, with 95% confidence, whether the data fit a normal distribution. Clearly state your hypotheses and show all working. ■

7.3.5 Chi-Square Test for Normality

The Shapiro–Wilk test was designed for use with small sample sizes. Although there is no hard-and-fast rule, a rule of thumb is that it is suitable when dealing with sample sizes of 50 or less. One alternative to the Shapiro–Wilk test that may be more powerful for larger sample sizes is the χ^2 test. In Section 6.5, we saw the use of the χ^2 test for testing hypotheses about categorical data. A slightly different form of the test can be used to test the goodness-of-fit of a sample against any expected distribution. We will demonstrate its use for testing against a normal distribution.

To illustrate the use of the χ^2 test, we introduce a new case study. A team of biomedical engineers has developed a technique for automatically estimating gestational age from a magnetic resonance (MR) scan of a fetus. They have tested their technique on 300 fetal MR scans for which the "gold standard" gestational age was known. Based on these data, they have computed the errors in gestational age estimation for their technique. These errors are summarized in Table 7.1. To perform further statistical analysis on the error figures, the team would like to know if their data are normally distributed or not. We will work to a 95% degree of confidence.

The null hypothesis for the χ^2 goodness-of-fit test is that there is no significant difference between the sample data and the expected distribution (in this case, a normal distribution). The alternative hypothesis is that there is a difference. To decide whether or not we can reject the null hypothesis, we need to compute the χ^2 test statistic Calc χ^2. In a similar way to the χ^2 tests that we saw in Section 6.5, the χ^2 goodness-of-fit test computes the test statistic by comparing observed frequencies with expected frequencies. This time, we compare observed frequencies of sample values within particular ranges (or *bins*) with those that would be expected if the sample were from a normal distribution with the same mean and standard deviation as the sample. This comparison is summarized in Table 7.2. The first column shows the bins (or ranges) of errors used (i.e. the same as in Table 7.1). The second column shows the probabilities of sample values from these bins (assuming that the sample was normally distributed). These probabilities can be computed from the areas under a normal distribution with the same mean and standard deviation as the sample (e.g. see Fig. 4.5B). Based on these probabilities and the sample size, we can compute expected frequencies E for each bin. These values are shown in the third column of the table. For example, the value for the < -10 bin is 3.39,

Table 7.1 Errors in MR-based gestational age estimation for 300 fetuses.

Error in gestational age estimation (days)	Number of cases
Less than -10	2
Between -10 and -5	36
Between -5 and 0	123
Between 0 and 5	97
Between 5 and 10	38
More than 10	4

Table 7.2 Computation of Calc χ^2 for the gestational age error data.

Gest. age error	Prob	E		O		$\frac{(O-E)^2}{E}$
<-10	0.0113	3.39	$\Big\}$38.09	2	$\Big\}$38	0.0002
≥ -10 and < -5	0.1157	34.7		36		
≥ -5 and < 0	0.3723	111.7		123		1.14
≥ 0 and < 5	0.373	111.9		97		2.29
≥ 5 and < 10	0.1163	34.89	$\Big\}$38.31	38	$\Big\}$42	0.36
≥ 10	0.0114	3.42		4		
Totals:	1.0	300.0		300		Calc $\chi^2 = 3.79$

which is equal to the probability 0.0113 multiplied by the sample size 300. The fourth column shows the observed frequencies O, which are reproduced from Table 7.1. Finally, the fifth column shows the χ^2 statistic for each row. This is computed as the square of the difference between the observed and expected frequencies divided by the expected frequency. The final test statistic, Calc χ^2, is the sum of all of these χ^2 statistics. Note that this is the same formula as we used for the χ^2 tests that we saw in Section 6.5, that is, Eq. (6.4), which is reproduced here for convenience:

$$\chi^2 = \sum \frac{(O - E)^2}{E}.$$

Note that the frequencies for the first two bins (<-10, ≥-10 and <-5) have been combined. We should always do this when the frequency of any bin is less than or equal to 5. In our case, the first bin (<-10) has both observed and expected frequencies that are less than or equal to 5. Therefore, we have to combine the first two bins to ensure that both expected and observed frequencies are greater than 5. We perform the same combination for the last two bins for the same reason.

After we have calculated our test statistic, we simply compare it to a critical value from Table A.5. To look up the critical value, we must know the number of degrees of freedom of the test. For a χ^2 goodness-of-fit test, the number of degrees of freedom is the number of bins minus 3. We subtract 3 because we already know that the sums of the expected and observed frequencies are the same, and we also know the mean and standard deviation of the distribution. For our example, we have 4 bins (after the first two and the last two have been combined). Therefore, we have $4 - 3 = 1$ degree of freedom. From Table A.5 we see that our critical value Tab χ^2 for a 0.05 significance level (i.e. 95% confidence) is equal to 3.841. Because Calc $\chi^2 = 3.79$ is not bigger than Tab $\chi^2 = 3.841$, we do not reject the null hypothesis that the data are from a normal distribution.

■ The Intuition. The Chi-Square Goodness-of-Fit Test

The intuition behind the χ^2 goodness-of-fit test is similar to that described for the χ^2 tests that we saw in Section 6.5. The χ^2 test statistic has a known distribution as shown in Fig. 6.4. The null hypothesis of normality is rejected when the statistic is large enough to go beyond the critical χ^2 value Tab χ^2 for the given significance level, that is, it becomes unlikely that we would get a value this large or larger by chance.   ■

■ Activity 7.4

O7.F   Resting heart rate data (in beats per minute, bpm) have been gathered from a cohort of 350 volunteers. The data are summarized in the table and histogram below.

Heart rate	Probability	Expected frequency, E	Observed frequency, O	$\frac{(O-E)^2}{E}$
<60	0.0096		3	
60–65	0.0238		12	
65–70	0.0594		19	
70–75	0.115		39	
75–80	0.1726		55	
80–85	0.2009		75	
85–90	0.1814		67	
90–95	0.127		47	
95–100	0.0689		16	
100–105	0.029		12	
105–110	0.0095		3	
>110	0.0029		2	
Totals:	1.0		350	Calc $\chi^2 =$

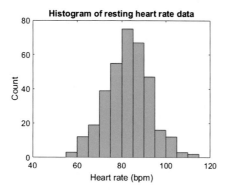

The mean heart rate is 82.9 bpm, and the standard deviation is 9.8 bpm. The table also shows the probabilities of the different heart rate bins based on a normal distribution with the same mean and standard deviation. The expected frequency and χ^2 test statistic columns have been left blank for you to fill in.

Use the values in the table to perform the χ^2 test by hand to test if the heart rate data come from a normal distribution. ∎

7.4 SHOULD WE USE A PARAMETRIC OR NONPARAMETRIC TEST?

We have now seen a number of different statistical hypothesis tests, both parametric and nonparametric. When making use of tests such as these, it is important to choose an appropriate test. This enables us to be sure that our conclusions are legitimate and also that we have used the maximum statistical power at our disposal. It can sometimes be difficult to choose between parametric and nonparametric tests, and in fact, statisticians often disagree about when certain tests can be applied and how to get the maximum power.

However, we can outline a few basic considerations that are worth remembering when choosing which test to apply. First, we should definitely choose a nonparametric test if we have ranked data (e.g. a grade such as A, B, C, etc.). We should also choose a nonparametric test if we know that our data were not drawn from a normal distribution. The following methods can be used to help us to decide if this is the case or not:

- Examine the data, for example, by using histograms or Q–Q plots.
- Use numerical measures, such as PPCC, skew, or z-values.
- Use a formal test of normality, such as the Shapiro–Wilk test or the χ^2 goodness-of-fit test.

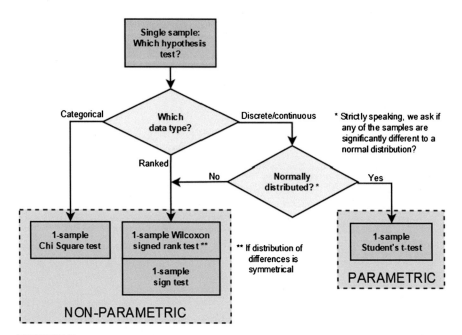

FIGURE 7.7
Summary of considerations when choosing an appropriate one sample hypothesis test.

■ Use information from other studies from the same population. Were these shown to be normally distributed?

■ Think about the causes of variation in our data: if the data are likely to be the result of lots of random factors then the resulting distribution is likely to be normal.

Figs. 7.7 and 7.8 present simplified flow diagrams summarizing some of the factors that should be considered when choosing a hypothesis test. Note that we only include in these diagrams the tests that we have covered in this book. In reality, there are many more tests to choose from, each with their own assumptions and strengths/weaknesses. But we hope that these diagrams will enable the interested reader to get started on analyzing and answering questions about their data and will act as a springboard from which to explore other types of test that may be suitable for their needs.

7.5 DOES IT MATTER IF WE USE THE WRONG TEST?

We have mentioned several times that parametric tests require the population variable(s) from which the sample data were drawn to be normally distributed. This is a widely applied and very useful rule. However, in hypothesis testing, we are typically interested in assessing a measure of central tendency, such as the mean. We saw in Chapter 4 that the central limit theorem states that the

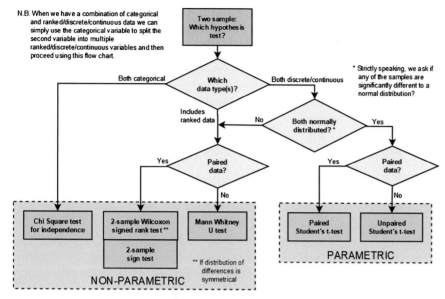

N.B. When we have a combination of categorical and ranked/discrete/continuous data we can simply use the categorical variable to split the second variable into multiple ranked/discrete/continuous variables and then proceed using this flow chart.

Two sample: Which hypothesis is test?

Both categorical

Which data type(s)?

Both discrete/continuous

* Strictly speaking, we ask if any of the samples are significantly different to a normal distribution?

Includes ranked data

No

Both normally distributed? *

Yes

Yes

Paired data?

Yes

Paired data?

No

No

Chi Square test for independence

2-sample Wilcoxon signed rank test **

Mann Whitney U test

Paired Student's t-test

Unpaired Student's t-test

2-sample sign test

** If distribution of differences is symmetrical

PARAMETRIC

NON-PARAMETRIC

FIGURE 7.8

Summary of considerations when choosing an appropriate two sample hypothesis test.

mean of a sample will *always* be approximately normally distributed so long as the sample size is large enough. So a legitimate question to ask is: if we are interested answering questions about the mean value, why not always use a parametric test? The answer to this question is that the assumption of normality is required to derive the formulation of the t-test. In reality the t-test does tend to be quite robust to nonnormally distributed data, so it may not matter that much if we apply a t-test with data whose distribution is only slightly different from a normal distribution. However, we should also bear in mind which measure of central tendency we are interested in – for highly skewed data, the mean is not an appropriate measure, and so the t-test should not be used.

Overall, it is certainly safest to only use a parametric test if we are sure that the variable(s) of interest are normally distributed. In fact, for large sample sizes, parametric and nonparametric tests will give similar results. However, for smaller sample sizes, the use of a parametric test on data from a clearly nonnormal population may result in an inaccurate result. The use of a nonparametric test on data from a clearly normal population will reduce the power of our statistics.

7.6 SUMMARY

To be able to apply an appropriate hypothesis test, it is important to be able to test assumptions about the distribution that the sample data were drawn from. One of the most common assumptions is that a sample was drawn from a normal distribution. A variety of visual and numerical techniques can be utilized to help us to decide if this assumption is valid.

Visual methods include plotting histograms or Q–Q plots. Q–Q plots illustrate the relationship between corresponding quantiles between two samples or between a sample and a theoretical distribution. A quantile is a value below which a certain proportion of the data values will lie. If the relationship between a sample's quantile values and those of a normal distribution is linear, then the sample is likely to have been drawn from a normal distribution.

Numerical methods include the probability plot correlation coefficient (PPCC), which is the correlation coefficient of the quantile values. A PPCC value of 1 indicates a linear relationship, and hence that the sample came from the theoretical distribution. Skew values can also be calculated, with a magnitude greater than 1 indicating a significant skew. z-values involve transforming the data to a standard normal distribution and enable us to assess the proportions of data values that lie beyond certain multiples of the standard deviation from the mean. These proportions can be compared against known values for a normal distribution.

The Shapiro–Wilk test and the chi-square (χ^2) test are formal tests, which can be used to test whether samples were likely to have been drawn from a normal distribution. The Shapiro–Wilk test is suitable for small samples, typically ≤ 50, whereas the χ^2 test is suitable for larger samples.

7.7 ASSESSING DATA DISTRIBUTIONS USING MATLAB

In this section, we detail the MATLAB functions that are provided for assessing the distribution of data samples. Where no built-in function is available, we provide basic implementations ourselves.

7.7.1 Visual Methods

Histograms:

```
histogram(x,nbins)
```

Produces a histogram from the array x. The optional parameter nbins specifies the number of bins to use in the histogram.

Q–Q Plot:

```
qqplot(x)
```

Displays a quantile–quantile plot of sample data x against a standard normal distribution.

7.7.2   Numerical Methods

Probability Plot Correlation Coefficient:

There is no built-in MATLAB function to compute the PPCC. The implementation given below will compute the PPCC of an array `data` against a standard normal distribution.

ppcc.m:

```
function coef = ppcc(data)
% compute probability plot correlation coefficient (PPCC)
% usage:
%   coef = ppcc(data)
%     data: sample data
%     coef: PPCC value

% make sure it's a column vector
data = data(:);

n=length(data);  % sample size
data=sort(data); % sort data

% compute PPCC
for i=1:n % loop over all the data values
    %calculate the fraction of data we need below
    % each quantile value
    frac = (i-0.5)/n;
    % calculate the quantile values from a standard
    % normal distribution, and save in an array
    normq(i) = norminv(frac);
end

coef = corr(data,normq'); % Pearson's r
% note because input is a column vector, while
% normq is a row vector we need to transpose
% one using '

end
```

Skew:

As noted in Chapter 1, the skew of a sample array x can be calculated in MATLAB using the following calculation:

```
3*(mean(x) - median(x))/std(x)
```

z-**values**:

```
z = zscore(x)
```

Compute the *z*-values of the sample data x.

Shapiro–Wilk Test:

There is no built-in function in MATLAB to perform the Shapiro–Wilk test. The basic implementation that we have provided below will perform the test at 0.05 significance for a maximum sample size of 10. See Section 7.8 for details of how to download a more flexible implementation.

shapiro_wilk_test.m:

```
function h = shapiro_wilk_test(d)
% perform Shapiro—Wilk test at 0.05 significance
% usage:
%    h = shapiro_wilk_test(d)
%       d: sample data
%       h: result: zero means do not reject null hypothesis
%                  that data are normal

% make sure it's a column vector
d = d(:);

% check sample size is valid
if length(d) > 10
    error('shapiro_wilk_test:  sample size must be <= 10');
end

% Shapiro—Wilk coefficients a for n<=10
swcoeff=[0.0000 0.7071 0.7071 0.6872 0.6646 ...
            0.6431 0.6233 0.6052 0.5888 0.5739; ...
            0.0000 0.0000 0.0000 0.1677 0.2413 ...
            0.2806 0.3031 0.3164 0.3244 0.3291; ...
            0.0000 0.0000 0.0000 0.0000 0.0000 ...
            0.0875 0.1401 0.1743 0.1976 0.2141; ...
            0.0000 0.0000 0.0000 0.0000 0.0000 ...
            0.0000 0.0000 0.0561 0.0947 0.1224; ...
            0.0000 0.0000 0.0000 0.0000 0.0000 ...
            0.0000 0.0000 0.0000 0.0000 0.0399];

% Shapiro—Wilk tabulated values for alpha=0.05 and n<=10
swtab=[0 0 0.767 0.748 0.762 0.788 0.803 0.818 0.829 0.842];

% sort data
ds = sort(d);

% compute b
n = length(ds);
s = std(ds);
b = 0;
for i=1:n/2
    b = b + (ds(n—i+1)—ds(i))*swcoeff(i,n);
end

% compute test statistic w
calcw = (b*b) / ((n—1)*s*s);
```

```
% find tabulated value w
tabw = swtab(n);

% compare calculated and tabulated w
% null hypothesis: data are from normal distribution
% alternative hypothesis: it's not
if (calcw > tabw)
    h = 0; % do not reject null hypothesis
else
    h = 1; % reject null hypthesis - data are not normal
end

end
```

Chi-Square Test for Normality:

```
[h, p] = chi2gof(x)
```

Performs a χ^2 goodness-of-fit test at 95% confidence for data sample x against a normal distribution. A return value of h$=1$ means that the null hypothesis that the sample is normally distributed is rejected, that is, the sample is not normally distributed. A return value of h$=0$ means that the null hypothesis cannot be rejected. The return value p is the *p*-value of the hypothesis test.

7.8 FURTHER RESOURCES

- The MATLAB Statistics and Machine Learning Toolbox documentation features a full list of functions available for performing other types of hypothesis test: https://mathworks.com/help/stats/hypothesis-tests-1.html
- A MATLAB script for performing the Shapiro–Wilk test is available for download from the Mathworks File Exchange: https://mathworks.com/matlabcentral/fileexchange/13964-shapiro-wilk-and-shapiro-francia-normality-tests

7.9 EXERCISES

Perform the following tasks, either by hand or using MATLAB, as specified.

■ **Exercise 7.1**

The contaminant level data for Professor A's new "Wonder 2" drug are contained in the file "profa_wonder2.txt", which is available from the book's web site. Use MATLAB to produce a Q–Q plot of these data against a standard normal distribution. O7.A

■ Exercise 7.2

O7.B   Use MATLAB to verify the PPCC figure of 0.9205 for Professor A's purity data given in Section 7.3.1.   ■

■ Exercise 7.3

O7.A   The MATLAB `qqplot` function can be used to produce a Q–Q plot of one sample against another or (if only one argument is provided) of one sample against a standard normal distribution. Write a new function that produces a Q–Q plot of a sample against a standard t-distribution with specified number of degrees of freedom. The function should take two arguments: the data sample (an array) and an integer representing the degrees of freedom. It does not need to return any value. The basic steps that your code should implement are:

   ■ Generate a (large) random sample from a standard t-distribution (i.e. with $\mu = 0$ and $\sigma = 1$) with the specified number of degrees of freedom.
   ■ Produce a Q–Q plot of the t-distribution sample against the sample provided as an argument.
   ■ Annotate the plot appropriately.

   Once you have written your function, use it to produce a Q–Q plot against an appropriate t-distribution for Professor A's "Wonder 2" drug contaminant level data.   ■

■ Exercise 7.4

O7.C   Use MATLAB to compute the skew of the "Wonder 2" drug contaminant level data.   ■

■ Exercise 7.5

O7.D   Use MATLAB to verify the computation of the z-values of the "Wonder 2" drug contaminant level data. You can check your results against the values given in Section 7.3.3.   ■

■ Exercise 7.6

O7.E   As part of a study on Alzheimer's disease patients, 8 patients were given a cognitive impairment test. The scores out of 20 were (high meaning impairment): (18.44 14.18 19.79 15.73 15.36 16.17 13.91 15.35). Perform a Shapiro–Wilk test to determine if the sample comes from a normal distribution. You can use MATLAB to do the calculations if you want, but you should follow the steps to apply the test by hand as outlined in Section 7.3.4.   ■

■ **Exercise 7.7**

In Activity 7.4, you performed a χ^2 goodness-of-fit test on volunteer heart rate data. The heart rate data are available to you through the book's web site as the file "hr_data.mat". Use MATLAB to perform the same χ^2 goodness-of-fit test to verify the result that you got in Activity 7.4.   ■

O7.F

■ **Exercise 7.8**

Image *segmentation* refers to the process of delineating the boundaries of regions of interest in an image. In medical imaging, segmentation can be useful for delineating organs or tumors to derive clinical measurements and assess disease. Segmentation can be performed manually using an interactive software tool. Manual segmentations are normally very accurate but can be very time-consuming to produce. Therefore, there is significant interest in developing automatic segmentation algorithms that can delineate regions of interest with no human interaction at all.

O7.G

A research team has developed a new technique for automatic liver segmentation from magnetic resonance (MR) images and wishes to compare the new approach to a comparative technique, which is considered to be the current state-of-the-art.

One way of assessing the similarity between segmentations is by computing a *Dice coefficient*. A Dice coefficient measures the degree of overlap between two segmentations and is a number between 0 and 1, with 0 representing no overlap and 1 representing full overlap.

To assess the accuracy of the liver segmentations produced by the new and comparative techniques, a junior doctor has manually segmented the livers from 35 MR scans. These manual segmentations are considered to be the "gold standard" segmentations. Dice coefficients have been computed between the segmentations produced by the new/comparative techniques and the gold standard.

These data are available to you in the file "segmentation.mat" from the book's web site, which contains the following variables:

■ `dice_new`: The Dice coefficients between the segmentations produced by the new technique and the gold standard segmentations.
■ `dice_comparative`: The Dice coefficients between the segmentations produced by the comparative technique and the gold standard segmentations.

Based on these data, use MATLAB to determine if the new segmentation technique is more accurate than the comparative technique. Be as thorough as possible in your data analysis and make sure that you choose and apply an appropriate hypothesis test to answer the question. Use a 95% degree of confidence.

FAMOUS STATISTICIAN: CARL FRIEDRICH GAUSS

This chapter's Famous Statistician is more of a general mathematician/scientist, but he made undoubted contributions that have greatly influenced the field of statistics. Carl Friedrich Gauss is sometimes referred to as the "Prince of Mathematicians". He had a remarkable influence in many fields of mathematics and science and is ranked as one of history's most influential mathematicians.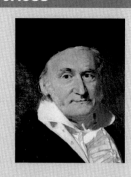

Gauss was born in 1777 to poor parents in Braunschweig, now part of Lower Saxony, Germany. He was a child prodigy and completed a major (and still influential today) work on number theory at the age of 21. Among his many achievements is his work on the normal (or Gaussian) distribution. This has proved very influential on the field of statistics and is central to the problems of estimating confidence intervals and testing hypotheses. Gauss was notoriously committed to his work, and one story goes that he was once interrupted in the middle of a problem and told that his wife was dying. He is reported to have said "Tell her to wait a moment till I'm done." Gauss himself died in Germany in 1855, aged 77.

CHAPTER 8

Inferential Statistics V: Multiple and Multivariate Hypothesis Testing

8.1 INTRODUCTION

In all of the hypothesis tests that we have seen in Chapters 5 and 6 of this book, there have been two significant limitations that have helped to simplify our analysis. First, we have only been asking a single question about the data. For example, does Professor A's "Wonder" drug have a lower contaminant level than Professor B's drug? Often, this is all that we want to do with inferential statistics. However, there are many cases in which we might want to ask multiple questions about our data at the same time or to analyze multiple "groups" of data. The second limitation has been that our data have consisted of single variables, that is, they have been *univariate* (see Section 1.2). Examples of univariate data that we have seen include the contaminant level in a drug sample or a subject's height. Both can be represented by a single number. Again, often this is sufficient, but there are cases in which we might want to analyze data represented by multiple values (i.e. they are *multivariate*). In fact, as we shall see, these two issues are related, and this chapter will introduce a number of techniques that can be applied in such situations.

Statistics for Biomedical Engineers and Scientists. https://doi.org/10.1016/B978-0-08-102939-8.00017-7

8.2 MULTIPLE HYPOTHESIS TESTING

We will deal first with the issue of asking multiple questions about our data. We first explain why we need to think about how to approach this situation, and then introduce a simple but widely used method for addressing the potential problem that is faced. After this, we deal with the related issue of asking questions about multiple groups of data.

8.2.1 Bonferroni's Correction

Suppose that we have a large scale database acquired from volunteers. The database contains multiple parameters such as the amount of exercise that the volunteers do, how much alcohol they drink, whether or not they smoke, how good their diet is, and so on. The database also contains metrics of cardiac health, such as the ejection fraction,[1] and we want to find out which of the parameters in the database are linked to cardiac health. To achieve this, we might want to ask multiple questions about our data. For instance:

- Do nonsmokers have higher ejection fractions than smokers?
- Do heavy drinkers have lower ejection fractions than nondrinkers?
- Do people with good diet have higher ejection fractions than those with poor diet?
- Do people who do a lot of exercise have higher ejection fractions than those who do not?

We do not know which, if any, of these questions will have a positive answer. We just want to learn about the influences on cardiac health by examining a number of different possibilities. How would we go about answering these questions? The obvious approach would be to perform an individual hypothesis test for each question that we want to ask, for example, we could split up the ejection fraction data into two groups according to the variable of interest (e.g. smoking, drinking, etc.) and test for a significant difference between the groups. However, let us think about what would happen if we did this. Recall from Section 5.2 that a type I error occurs when we reject the null hypothesis when in reality there is no difference in the population variable. If we are working to a 95% degree of confidence, there is a 5% chance of getting a type I error *if we perform a single hypothesis test*. This is considered to be an acceptably small probability. But what if we perform, say, 100 hypothesis tests. In this case, we would expect to get 5 type I errors, that is, we would reject the null hypothesis and find a significant difference even though none exists 5 times. If we did 1000 hypothesis tests, then we would expect to get 50 type I errors, and so on.

---

[1]The proportion of blood pumped out of the heart's left ventricle in each heart beat. A low value can be a sign of heart disease.

So we can see that the more questions we ask about our data, the more wrong answers we are likely to get. This is clearly not a desirable situation.

Bonferroni's correction is a simple adjustment that we can make when performing multiple hypothesis tests that tries to ensure that we do not increase the chance of getting at least one type I error. Recall that hypothesis tests such as the Student's t-test return a p-value that represents the probability of the sample distribution (or a more extreme one) occurring by chance if the null hypothesis were true. The null hypothesis states that there is no difference between the population variables of interest and we reject the null hypothesis if the p-value is less than our critical value, which for a single test is equal to the significance level α, for example, 0.05 for a 95% degree of confidence. With Bonferroni's correction, we adjust the critical value for each test to α/m, where m is the number of tests being performed. By making this adjustment, the *familywise error rate* (the chance of getting at least one type I error) is not increased as a result of performing multiple tests.

For example, let us return to our large-scale database example. Suppose that we perform the four hypothesis tests listed above and that the resulting p-values are 0.04, 0.1, 0.02, and 0.01. Without performing Bonferroni's correction and working to a 95% degree of confidence, we would reject the null hypothesis (and answer "yes" to the questions being asked) in three of the four cases, since three of the p-values are less than $\alpha = 0.05$. However, after applying Bonferroni's correction the critical value is adjusted to $0.05/4 = 0.0125$, so we now only reject the null hypothesis in one case, that is, the last question, which returned a p-value of 0.01.

■ **The Intuition. Bonferroni's Correction**

It seems intuitive that there is a greater likelihood of a type I error if we do more tests, but what exactly is the chance of at least one type I error occurring? For a single test, that is easy – it is equal to the significance level α. For two tests, it becomes $1 - (1 - \alpha)^2$. So for $\alpha = 0.05$ (i.e. a 95% degree of confidence), the chance of at least one type I error in two tests is $1 - 0.95^2 = 0.0975$. For three tests, it is $1 - 0.95^3 = 0.1426$, and so on. In general, the chance of at least one type I error for m tests is

$$P_{\text{type I}} = 1 - (1 - \alpha)^m. \tag{8.1}$$

Fig. 8.1A shows the variation of $P_{\text{type I}}$ as the number of tests increases. By the time we reach 20 tests the chance is already 0.6415, or 64%.

If we apply Bonferroni's correction, then the critical value is reduced as a function of the number of tests, so the chance of a type I error becomes

$$P_{\text{type I,Bonferroni}} = 1 - (1 - \alpha/m)^m. \tag{8.2}$$

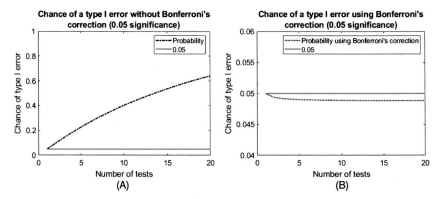

FIGURE 8.1

The chance of at least one type I error occurring in multiple hypothesis tests at 0.05 significance: (A) without Bonferroni's correction, (B) with Bonferroni's correction. Note the different scales on the y-axes.

The only difference between Eqs. (8.1) and (8.2) is the division of α by m. Fig. 8.1B shows the variation of $P_{\text{type I,Bonferroni}}$ with the number of tests. We can see that the chance of at least one type I error is never higher than the significance level for a single test, that is, $\alpha = 0.05$. ∎

■ **Activity 8.1**

O8.A   Functional magnetic resonance imaging (fMRI) uses MR scanning to measure brain activity by detecting changes associated with blood oxygenation. A team of neuroscientists is investigating the links between regional brain activity and performance of a specific task. Fifteen volunteers were scanned, and their fMRI activity levels were computed. The activity levels consist of a single variable representing the level of oxygenation within a localized brain region, and they were computed whilst the volunteers were performing the task and also whilst they were resting. The levels were recorded for the following brain regions: *frontal lobe, parietal lobe, temporal lobe, occipital lobe*, and *cerebellum*. Student's *t*-tests between the task and rest activity levels over all volunteers resulted in the following *p*-values for the five brain regions: 0.011, 0.0037, 0.0011, 0.1234, and 0.1153.

Working to a 95% degree of confidence, state which of the five brain regions had a different level of activity whilst performing the task. ∎

8.2.2   Analysis of Variance (ANOVA)

A related issue to multiple hypothesis testing is the case where we have multiple "groups" of data, which represent the same variable of interest. For example, we may measure the blood pressures of a number of subjects and want to

Table 8.1 Mean and variance of MMSE score differences for four groups of Alzheimer's disease patients based on treatment strategy. A negative number indicates a decline in cognitive ability.

Treatment strategy	MMSE score difference	
	Mean	*Variance*
None	−3.6	3.17
Physical exercise	−2.72	4.21
Mental stimulation	−2.32	3.56
Drug	−3.2	5.58

group them according to diet (*good*, *acceptable*, and *poor*). In this case the data are univariate, since we are only concerned with analyzing a single variable (blood pressure), but we have three samples representing the different dietary groups. Analysis of variance (ANOVA) is a technique designed for answering questions about such groups of data.

ANOVA attempts to answer the specific question of whether all groups have the same mean or at least one pair of group means is significantly different. Therefore, in contrast to Bonferroni's correction, ANOVA is a single test that assesses multiple sample groups. But the aim of ANOVA is the same as that of Bonferroni's correction – to avoid increasing the chance of at least one type I error. Note also that the name ANOVA (analysis of *variance*) may seem strange at first as we are interested in means not variances, but as we will see, we do this by looking at variances.

We will use a case study to illustrate the use of ANOVA. A research programme is investigating the efficacy of different treatment strategies for Alzheimer's disease. Alzheimer's disease is a condition that causes a progressive decline in cognitive ability. One way of measuring cognitive ability is by using the Mini Mental State Examination (MMSE). The MMSE is a test containing 30 questions, and so results in a score between 0–30, with a lower score (typically less than 24) indicating some level of cognitive impairment. The research programme is investigating four different strategies for controlling cognitive decline in a cohort of Alzheimer's disease patients: doing nothing, a programme of physical exercise, a programme of mental stimulation, and drug treatment.

100 early stage Alzheimer's disease patients have been recruited and split randomly into four groups of 25. Each group undertook one of the four treatment strategies. MMSE scores were recorded for each patient before and after the treatment period, and the MMSE differences were computed. This difference is the variable of interest, and a negative difference indicates a decline in cognitive ability. We want to know if there is any difference between the strategies in terms of controlling cognitive decline. The results of the study are summarized in Table 8.1.

Before proceeding to the numerical calculations of the ANOVA test, we first introduce some terminology. In the context of ANOVA, a *factor* refers to an independent variable that is used to split our sample data into groups. We are typically interested in analyzing the effect of the factor on the (dependent) variable of interest. For our case study, the factor is the treatment strategy, and the dependent variable is the MMSE score difference. A factor typically has a number of *levels*, which refers to the values that the independent variable can take. For us, the levels are the different treatments, that is, *none, physical exercise, mental stimulation,* and *drug*. If we have only one factor (as we do in the Alzheimer's disease example), then we refer to the test as a "one-way ANOVA"; if we have two factors, then it is a "two-way ANOVA."

Now we will perform the one-way ANOVA test for our case study. ANOVA is a hypothesis test, so we follow the checklist for hypothesis testing that we introduced in Section 5.2:

- *Examine the data.* Summary statistics are given in Table 8.1, and histograms of the group samples are shown in Fig. 8.2.
- *Form null and alternative hypotheses and choose a degree of confidence.* The null hypothesis for ANOVA is that all groups have the same mean. The alternative hypothesis is that at least one pair of group means is significantly different. Note that the null/alternative hypotheses do not specify which two means are different, just whether any two are different. Therefore ANOVA cannot tell us this information. We will work to a 95% degree of confidence.

Next, we need to compute a test statistic. To explain the test statistic, we first need to understand a bit more about how ANOVA operates. ANOVA involves making two different estimates of the population variance σ^2 (hence the name, analysis of *variance*). One of these estimates is sensitive to differences in mean between the groups, and the other is not. Therefore, *if all groups have the same mean, then the two estimates of variance will be approximately the same.* If they do not have the same mean, then they will be different.

The two estimates of variance are known as the mean square error (MSE), which is based on differences between sample values *within* groups, and the mean square between (MSB), which is based on differences in sample means *between* groups. We now explain how each of these is calculated and used to compute our test statistic.

To compute MSE, we assume that all groups have the same variance, and so the population variance can be estimated by simply taking the means of the sample variances from each group:

$$MSE = \frac{1}{k} \sum_{i=1}^{k} s_i^2, \tag{8.3}$$

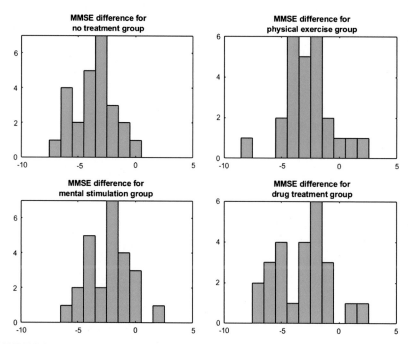

FIGURE 8.2

Histograms for the Mini Mental State Examination (MMSE) score differences for four groups of Alzheimer's patients: no treatment, physical exercise, mental stimulation, drug treatment.

where k is the number of groups, and s_i^2 represents the sample variance for group i.

For example, for our Alzheimer's disease example, the four group variances as shown in Table 8.1 are 3.17, 4.21, 3.56, and 5.58. The mean of these values is 4.13, so this is our value for MSE. Note that because this estimate is based only on group *variances* and not *means*, it is not sensitive to any differences in mean between the groups.

The second estimate of the population variance (MSB) comes from multiplying the variance of the sample means by the group sample size (for the moment, we assume that all groups have the same size):

$$MSB = n \times \left(\frac{1}{k-1} \sum_{i=1}^{k} (\bar{x}_i - \bar{x})^2 \right)$$
(8.4)

where n is the group sample size, $\bar{x}_i$ is the sample mean of group i and $\bar{x}$ is the overall sample mean (i.e. of the pooled groups). Note that the rightmost term (in brackets) is the variance of the sample means (see Section 1.5).

For our Alzheimer's disease example, we have a group sample size of 25, and the group sample means are -3.6, -2.72, -2.32, and -3.2. Therefore, using

Eq. (8.4), we compute the MSB to be 7.79. Note that MSB is based on group *mean* values, so any difference in group means will cause MSB to overestimate the true population variance.

Now we have values for our two population variance estimates, MSE and MSB. We also know that if MSB is larger than MSE, then it may be a sign that the group means are not equal. This may also happen by chance. So how much larger should MSB be in order to reject the null hypothesis? The mathematical formulation for this was one of the many contributions to the field of statistics of this chapter's Famous Statistician, Ronald Fisher. The details are beyond the scope of this book, but the statistic of interest is named after Fisher and is called the F statistic. It is equal to the ratio of MSB to MSE.

Returning to our example, we have $F = \text{MSB}/\text{MSE} = 7.79/4.13 = 1.89$. Is this too large? We determine this by comparing it to a critical F value from a table (see Tables A.8 and A.9 in the Appendix). To look up the critical value, we need two degrees of freedom values, one for MSE and one for MSB. MSE is an average of k variances (where k is the number of groups), each with $n - 1$ degrees of freedom, so the total degrees of freedom for MSE is $k(n - 1) = N - k$, where N is the total number of samples over all groups (i.e. $N = k \times n$). Since MSB is computed from the k group means, we have $k - 1$ degrees of freedom. For the Alzheimer's disease data, we have $n = 25$, $k = 4$, and $N = 100$, so we have 3 degrees of freedom for MSB and 96 degrees of freedom for MSE. From the tables we can see that our critical value is 2.699. Therefore, if our calculated F statistic is greater than 2.698, then we reject the null hypothesis. However, our calculated F statistic is 1.89, so we cannot conclude with 95% confidence that there is at least one pair of means that is different.

■ The Intuition. ANOVA

We know that ANOVA is based on estimating the overall population variance σ^2 in two different ways, MSE and MSB. If the group means are equal (i.e. the null hypothesis is true), then both should give approximately the same result, but if they are not equal, then MSB will overestimate σ^2. Why is this?

MSE is the average of the group sample variances. Therefore, assuming that all variances are approximately equal, it should be clear that this will be a reasonable estimate of σ^2.

But what about MSB? We know that the standard deviation of the distribution of mean values estimated from a sample (i.e. the standard error of the mean) is $\sigma/\sqrt{n}$ (see Section 4.6), where n is the sample size. The variance is simply the square of the standard deviation, so the variance of the distribution of mean values is: $\sigma^2_{\text{mean}} = \sigma^2/n$. Rearranging this formula gives $\sigma^2 = n \times \sigma^2_{\text{mean}}$. Therefore, using the variance of the group sample means

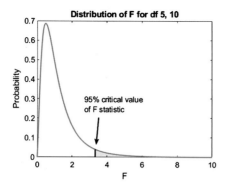

FIGURE 8.3

The distribution of the F statistic for ANOVA (degrees of freedom 5 and 10) and the critical value for a 95% degree of confidence.

s_{mean}^2 as an estimate of σ_{mean}^2, we can estimate σ^2 by

$$\sigma^2 \approx n \times s_{mean}^2. \qquad (8.5)$$

This is equivalent to the formula for MSB that we introduced in Eq. (8.4).

Now, if the population group means are not equal, then MSE will still estimate σ^2 because differences in population means do not affect variances. However, MSB will overestimate σ^2 because differences between population means will lead to differences between sample means and hence to a larger variance of the mean. Therefore, the larger the differences between sample means, the larger the MSB.

Fig. 8.3 shows the distribution of the F statistic for 5 and 10 degrees of freedom. The figure also shows the critical value for a 95% degree of confidence. If the calculated F statistic exceeds this value, then there is a less than 5% chance that this would have happened by chance if the null hypothesis were true.

Finally, note the assumptions of ANOVA: all groups' populations should be normally distributed and have the same variance. ∎

■ Activity 8.2

The New York Heart Association (NYHA) functional classification is a way of classifying heart failure patients based on the severity of their symptoms. There are four NYHA classes, denoted by the numbers 1 to 4, in increasing order of severity, as summarized in the following table.   *O8.B*

Class	Description
1	Patients with cardiac disease but resulting in no limitation of physical activity.
2	Patients with cardiac disease resulting in slight limitation of physical activity.
3	Patients with cardiac disease resulting in marked limitation of physical activity.
4	Patients with cardiac disease resulting in inability to carry on any physical activity without discomfort.

The NYHA class is typically determined by consultation with a cardiologist. A team of biomedical engineers is investigating more objective ways of measuring the severity of heart failure. One measure under investigation is the peak ejection rate (PER). This measures the left ventricular volume gradient of the ejection phase of the cardiac cycle.

A cohort of 40 heart failure patients has been identified, of which 10 patients were in each of the four NYHA classes. The PER was measured for each patient from echocardiography images using automated software. These data are summarized in the following table.

NYHA class	PER (ml/s)	
	Mean	Variance
1	263.24	80.49
2	250.17	119.35
3	249.0	122.8
4	246.29	105.7
Variance	57.03	

Perform an ANOVA test by hand to determine, with 95% confidence, whether any pair of mean PER values is significantly different. ∎

ANOVA With Unequal Sample Sizes

The formulation given above assumed that the sample sizes within each group were the same. Another way of saying this is that the groups were "balanced". ANOVA can also be applied with "unbalanced" groups (i.e. samples with different sizes), but the calculations by hand get a little more complicated. We now briefly outline the formulation for ANOVA with unbalanced classes.

First, we consider the definition for MSE. Previously, we just averaged the group sample variances. If the group sample sizes are different, then we need to weight their contributions to the overall variance estimate accordingly. To do this, we calculate the sum of squared differences of the means, weighted by the sample sizes, and then divide by the MSE degrees of freedom:

$$SSE = \sum_{i=1}^{k} n_i (\bar{x}_i - \bar{x})^2,$$

$$MSE = SSE/df_{MSE}, \qquad (8.6)$$

where k is the number of groups, n_i is the sample size of group i, $\bar{x}_i$ is the sample mean of group i, $\bar{x}$ is the overall sample mean (i.e. of all groups pooled together), and df_{MSE} is the MSE degrees of freedom, that is, $N - k$. Using this formulation, groups with a larger sample size are weighted more highly when computing the variance estimate. But note that Eqs. (8.6) and (8.3) are equivalent if the sample sizes are equal.

For MSB, in the case of equal sample sizes, we multiplied the group sample size by the variance of the group means. If the groups have different sample sizes, then we need to first compute the sum of squared differences to the group mean for each group, sum all of these, and then divide by the degrees of freedom:

$$SSB = \sum_{i=1}^{k}\sum_{j=1}^{n_i}(x_{i,j} - \bar{x}_i)^2,$$
$$MSB = SSB/df_{MSB}, \qquad (8.7)$$

where $x_{i,j}$ are the individual sample values in group i, $\bar{x}_i$ is the sample mean of group i, n_i is the sample size of group i, and df_{MSB} is the MSB degrees of freedom, that is, $k - 1$. Again, note that Eqs. (8.7) and (8.4) are equivalent if the sample sizes are equal.

In reality, applying the simplified formulation when we have unbalanced groups is often not a problem. Furthermore, if we use automated tools such as MATLAB (see Section 8.6), then the correct formulation will be automatically applied.

8.3   MULTIVARIATE HYPOTHESIS TESTING

We now move on to the problem of *multivariate* hypothesis testing. Recall that multivariate means that we measure or record multiple variables for each "individual". For example, in the large-scale database we introduced in Section 8.2, for each volunteer, we recorded whether they smoked or not, and information about alcohol consumption, diet, exercise, and cardiac health. All of these can be thought of as different variables, and so the data as a whole are multivariate. However, in Section 8.2, *each question we asked was based on univariate data*, that is, only ejection fraction values (for different subsets of the sample) were analyzed in the hypothesis tests. For instance, we compared the ejection fractions of smokers and nonsmokers. Sometimes we are interested in asking questions about true multivariate data in a single test. As an example, we might want to assess multiple indicators of cardiac health rather than just ejection fraction, such as ejection fraction, peak strain,[2] and peak ejection rate.[3] What can we do in such cases?

The naive approach would be to simply perform multiple univariate tests. In the example given above, we could perform one (univariate) test to compare ejection fractions, one to compare peak strains, and one to compare peak ejection rates. However, we know from Section 8.2.1 that the more tests we perform, the greater will be the chance of at least one type I error occurring. We prefer to avoid increasing this chance, so performing multiple tests in this way is not a good choice.

Could we just perform multiple univariate tests and apply Bonferroni's correction? Yes, we could, but some differences may only be apparent when looking at multiple variables, and not just single variables. For example, it may be that differences in cardiac health only become apparent when examining more than one indicator, but are not apparent by looking at any single one. Performing multiple univariate tests would miss such differences. Therefore we need alternative methods. This section presents some common techniques that can be applied when performing hypothesis tests on multivariate data.

8.3.1 Hotelling's T^2 Test

Hotelling's T^2 test is a generalization of the Student's t-test to multivariate data. Therefore, it is a parametric test and assumes normally distributed data. More specifically, it assumes that the data were drawn from a *multivariate normal distribution*. A multivariate normal distribution is essentially a generalization of the univariate normal distribution (see Section 4.4.1) to more than one variable.

We will illustrate the test using the case of testing a single sample against expected values (i.e. similar to Section 5.5 for the t-test). First, we form our hypotheses. The null hypothesis is that there is no difference between our (multivariate) sample mean and the expected mean. The alternative hypothesis is that there is a difference.

To compute the test statistic for Hotelling's T^2 test, we first compute a T^2 value defined as

$$T^2 = n\, (\bar{\mathbf{x}} - \boldsymbol{\mu})^T\, C^{-1}\, (\bar{\mathbf{x}} - \boldsymbol{\mu}), \tag{8.8}$$

where n is the sample size, $\bar{\mathbf{x}}$ is the multivariate sample mean (i.e. a column vector), $\boldsymbol{\mu}$ is the column vector of expected values, and C is the sample *covariance matrix* (see Section 2.3.2).

---

[2]The maximum deformation of the ventricular myocardium during the cardiac cycle.
[3]The left ventricular volume gradient of the ejection phase.

For example, if the sample x contained p variables, then we would have

$$\mathbf{x} = \begin{bmatrix} x_1 \\ x_2 \\ \vdots \\ x_p \end{bmatrix}$$

and

$$\bar{\mathbf{x}} = \begin{bmatrix} \bar{x}_1 \\ \bar{x}_2 \\ \vdots \\ \bar{x}_p \end{bmatrix},$$

where $\bar{x}_1, \ldots, \bar{x}_p$ are the means of the corresponding elements of x across the sample. The definition of the covariance matrix was presented in Eq. (2.3) and is reproduced here for convenience:

$$C = \frac{1}{n-1} \sum_{i=1}^{n} (\mathbf{x}_i - \bar{\mathbf{x}})(\mathbf{x}_i - \bar{\mathbf{x}})^T . \tag{8.9}$$

Here, the subscript i represents the sample index, and n is again the sample size.

Looking at Eq. (8.8), we can see that large differences between the sample mean and the expected values will lead to a high value of T^2.

Eq. (8.8) is known as *Hotelling's* T^2 and is named after its inventor Harold Hotelling, who published the mathematical formulation of the test back in 1931 [8]. The test statistic for Hotelling's T^2 test is computed from the T^2 value as follows

$$F = \frac{n-p}{p(n-1)} T^2 \tag{8.10}$$

where p is the number of variables, and n is the sample size. Importantly, *it can be shown that the test statistic F follows an F-distribution (see Section 8.2.2) with p and n − p degrees of freedom.* A high value of F indicates a larger difference between the sample data and the expected values (because F is a scaled version of T^2). Because we know the distribution of F, we can use the critical values from Tables A.8 and A.9 to determine how large F should be in order to reject the null hypothesis. When using the tables, we need the degrees of freedom, which, as stated before, are p and $n - p$.

Let us illustrate the use of this test with an example. A study is investigating possible links between diet and depression. A group of 10 patients suffering from depression have been recruited, and four daily dietary intake values have been recorded for each patient: *selenium, vitamin D, omega-3 fatty acids,* and *zinc*. The recommended daily intakes for these are: selenium = 35 µg, vitamin D = 10 µg, omega-3 = 250 mg and zinc = 15 mg. We want to know if the patient cohort have significantly different dietary intakes to the recommended values.

The data for the 10 patients are presented in Table 8.2, which also shows the mean values for each variable. We want to compare these mean values with the expected values from the recommended daily intake figures. Our null hypothesis is that there is no difference between the two, and the alternative hypothesis is that there is a difference. We will work to a 95% degree of confidence.

Now we will compute our test statistic. First, to compute T^2, Eq. (8.8) needs the sample covariance matrix. Using the data in the table and Eq. (2.3), we can compute this to be

$$C = \begin{bmatrix} 42.3 & 3.03 & 34.86 & 8.04 \\ 3.03 & 24.79 & 35.01 & 10.95 \\ 34.86 & 35.01 & 187.05 & -4.23 \\ 8.04 & 10.95 & -4.23 & 20.44 \end{bmatrix}.$$

We also know the mean of the sample $\bar{x}$ (this is the bottom row of values in Table 8.2), μ is the vector of expected values $[35\ 10\ 250\ 15]^T$, and $n = 10$ is the sample size. Therefore, using Eq. (8.8), we compute $T^2 = 19.58$. This value, together with $n = 10$ and $p = 4$ (the number of variables), is used in Eq. (8.10) to compute our test statistic $F = 3.26$. To look up the critical F value, we find the degrees of freedom $p = 4$ and $n - p = 6$. From Table A.8 we see that our critical value for 4 and 6 degrees of freedom is 4.534. As 3.26 is not greater than 4.534, we cannot reject the null hypothesis, so we cannot show that there is any significant difference between the dietary intake of the patients and the recommended values.

■ **The Intuition. Hotelling's T^2 Test**

To understand Hotelling's T^2 test, we first return to the univariate case. Recall that the Student's t-test is based on the t statistic, which was defined in Eq. (5.1):

$$t = \frac{\bar{x} - \mu}{s/\sqrt{n}},$$

where $\bar{x}$ is the (univariate) sample mean, μ is the expected mean value, n is the sample size, and s is the sample standard deviation. This computes the difference between the sample mean and the expected mean in terms of the number of standard errors of the mean. Squaring both sides and rearranging

Table 8.2 Data from the study into the links between diet and depression.

| Patient no. | Daily dietary intake | | | |
	Serenium (μg)	Vitamin D (μg)	Omega-3 fatty acids (mg)	Zinc (mg)
1	30.21	4.57	243.7	16.39
2	34.8	16.16	274.4	12.21
3	34.54	17.65	259.67	23.08
4	21.02	5.72	239.51	7.83
5	24.56	8.85	254.89	12.36
6	20.59	16.85	235.83	18.09
7	32.49	6.84	251.23	11.72
8	20.95	15.87	271.98	15.07
9	37.91	12.28	256.98	17.62
10	25.96	9.22	237.61	20.03
Mean:	**28.3**	**11.4**	**252.58**	**15.44**

results in

$$t^2 = n\,(\bar{x} - \mu)\,(s^2)^{-1}\,(\bar{x} - \mu),$$

where s^2 is the sample variance.

Generalizing this to the multivariate case, the corresponding equation can be shown to be

$$T^2 = n\,(\bar{\mathbf{x}} - \boldsymbol{\mu})^T\,C^{-1}\,(\bar{\mathbf{x}} - \boldsymbol{\mu}),$$

where $\bar{\mathbf{x}}$ is now the multivariate sample mean, $\boldsymbol{\mu}$ is the vector of expected values, and C is the covariance matrix. This was presented earlier as Eq. (8.8), and the similarity with the univariate version is apparent.

The key to understanding Hotelling's T^2 test is that when we square a t-distributed (multivariate) random variable with p values and $n - 1$ degrees of freedom, the result is an F-distributed random variable with p and $n - p$ degrees of freedom. The mathematics underpinning this finding were described by Harold Hotelling in his original 1931 paper [8]. It was also shown that when the null hypothesis of the test is true (i.e. the sample mean is equal to the expected mean), we have the following approximation:

$$T^2 \approx \frac{p(n - 1)}{n - p}\,F_{p,n-p},$$

where $F_{p,n-p}$ represents the F-distribution with p and $n - p$ degrees of freedom. Rearranging this formula gives the equation for the F statistic from

Eq. (8.10):

$$F = \frac{n - p}{p(n - 1)} T^2.$$

As for the ANOVA test, the critical values represent values beyond which the area under the F-distribution is 5%. ∎

■ Activity 8.3

O8.C
A cohort of 20 volunteers has been recruited to take part in an evaluation of a new drug. The investigating team would like to be sure that the cohort have certain blood serum levels that are typical of the population as a whole. The table below shows the constituents measured from the volunteers together with their typical population values.

Constituent	Typical level
Calcium	10 mg/dL
Magnesium	2.8 mg/dL
Phosphorous	3.8 mg/dL
Bilirubin	1.0 mg/dL
Albumin	4.5 g/dL

To determine whether the cohort have typical blood serum levels, the team would like to perform a Hotelling's T^2 test. The T^2 statistic has been calculated from the data to be 12.84. What is the result of the test? ∎

Two Sample Hotelling's T^2 Test

The formulation of Hotelling's T^2 test described before was for testing a single sample against expected values. The test can be extended to the two-sample case in a similar way to the Student's t-test.

For two-sample *paired* data, we simply compute the differences between the paired sample data and use a one-sample test against expected values of zeros for all variables. This is exactly the same approach as we took when extending the t-test to two-sample paired data in Section 5.7. The degrees of freedom for the test are therefore p and $n - p$ as for the one-sample case.

For two-sample *unpaired* data, things are a little more complicated. As we have two samples now and each has its own covariance matrix, we need to calculate a combined covariance matrix as follows:

$$C = \frac{(n_1 - 1)C_1 + (n_2 - 1)C_2}{n_1 + n_2 - 2}, \tag{8.11}$$

where n_1 and n_2 are the sample sizes of data sets 1 and 2, and C_1 and C_2 are their covariance matrices. The equations for T^2 and F also change slightly to reflect the different sample sizes:

$$T^2 = \left(\frac{n_1 n_2}{n_1 + n_2}\right)(\bar{\mathbf{x}}_1 - \bar{\mathbf{x}}_2)^T C^{-1}(\bar{\mathbf{x}}_1 - \bar{\mathbf{x}}_2) \tag{8.12}$$

and

$$F = \frac{n_1 + n_2 - p - 1}{p(n_1 + n_2 - 2)} T^2. \tag{8.13}$$

The degrees of freedom to use for looking up the critical F value are now p and $n_1 + n_2 - p - 1$.

8.3.2 Multivariate Analysis of Variance (MANOVA)

To continue our discussion of multivariate hypothesis testing, let us return to the Alzheimer's disease example that we introduced in Section 8.2.2 when describing the ANOVA test. Recall that we recorded the differences in scores for the Mini Mental State Examination (MMSE) before and after treatment with one of four different treatment options. Therefore, for each subject, we had one variable, so the data were *univariate*, but we had four *groups* of data. Now suppose that, as well as the MMSE score differences, we also record the differences in scores for two alternative measures of cognitive function:

- *ADAS-cog*, the Alzheimer's Disease Assessment Scale – cognitive subscale. This is primarily a test of language and memory, and it is commonly used in assessment of Alzheimer's disease. The scores range from 0–70, with higher scores indicating greater cognitive impairment.
- *SIB*, the Severe Impairment Battery. This is another measure used in evaluating treatment response in Alzheimer's disease, and scores range from 0–100, with lower scores indicating greater cognitive impairment.

Now we have three variables for each subject (i.e. *multivariate* data), representing the differences in the three scores before and after treatment. Note that we cannot use Hotelling's T^2 test because we have more than two groups of data. So we need a version of ANOVA that can be used for multivariate data.

MANOVA (multivariate analysis of variance) is a generalization of ANOVA to multivariate data. The mathematical formulation of MANOVA is considerably more complex than that of ANOVA, and we do not attempt to go into it in detail in this book. By far the easiest way to apply MANOVA is to use an automated tool such as MATLAB (see Section 8.6). For more mathematical details, the interested reader is referred to the links for further reading in Section 8.7.

Here, we just note that even though the calculations involved are more complex, the basic principle behind them remains similar to ANOVA. Like ANOVA, MANOVA works by analyzing the variation in the data, but whereas ANOVA uses *variance*, MANOVA uses *covariance*. Recall from Sections 2.3.1 and 2.3.2 that covariance measures the joint variability of two variables, and the covariance matrix represents all variances and covariances between a number of variables. So, whereas in ANOVA we used calculations of sums of squares (i.e. SSE and SSB; see Section 8.2.2), in MANOVA these become matrices containing sums of squares and also sums of products.

The assumptions of MANOVA are also similar to those of ANOVA, but they are generalized to multivariate data. First, the data should be normally distributed, but now that the data are multivariate, we assume a multivariate normal distribution. Second, whereas ANOVA assumes a common variance between groups, MANOVA assumes a common covariance.

Due to the complexity of the calculations, it is rare to apply a MANOVA test by hand, and so we return to this test when discussing the use of MATLAB in Section 8.6.

8.4 WHICH TEST SHOULD WE USE?

We have now seen a number of different tests that can be used when we have multiple variables or want to test multiple hypotheses. When dealing with multiple and multivariate hypothesis testing, we can identify a number of different situations, and these are summarized in Table 8.3.

First, we either have two *groups* of data or we have more than two groups. The number of groups is related to the number of questions we want to ask about the data. For instance, in the case of Professor A's contaminant level data from Section 5.7.2, we had two groups of data, those from Professor A's technique and those from Professor B's technique. The only question we asked then was whether the group means were different or the same. In the example introduced in Section 8.2 about the large-scale database, we had more than two groups of data: we had ejection fractions for smokers, ejection fractions for nonsmokers, ejection fractions for heavy drinkers, and so on. So we were able to ask multiple questions about our data. However, our data were still univariate (i.e. just ejection fraction), so we applied Bonferroni's correction. In Section 8.2.2, we also had more than two groups of univariate data (i.e. MMSE score differences for different treatments), but we were only interested in asking a single question: do the groups have the same mean? So we applied an ANOVA test.

The second distinction we can make is what data we have in each group, that is, do we have univariate or multivariate data? In the case of both the large-scale database and Professor A's new drug, we had univariate data (ejection fraction and the contaminant level). In Sections 8.3.1 and 8.3.2, we had multivariate data in the form of multiple dietary intake values and multiple measures of cognitive function. We applied a Hotelling's T^2 test in Section 8.3.1 because

Table 8.3 A summary of which test can be applied depending on the number of groups and the number of variables within each group.

No. of groups of data	Number of variables in each group	
	Univariate	*Multivariate*
2	Student's t-test (see Section 5.7)	Hotelling's T^2 (see Section 8.3.1)
>2	Bonferroni's correction (see Section 8.2.1), ANOVA (see Section 8.2.2)	MANOVA (see Section 8.3.2)

we had two groups of data and a MANOVA test in Section 8.3.2 because we had more than two groups.

As always in statistics, it is important to choose the right test for the type of data and situation that we have, and Table 8.3 can be a useful reference for thinking about which test to apply.

■ **Activity 8.4**

For each of the following scenarios, state how many groups of data there are, what type of data there are (univariate/multivariate), and what hypothesis test you would apply. You can assume that all data are normally distributed.

O8.E

1. A study is investigating links between diet and intelligence. A group of volunteers has been recruited, and all have taken IQ tests. In addition, all volunteers took a blood test to measure levels of a range of different vitamins and minerals. Based on the measured levels, for each vitamin/mineral, the volunteers were classed as normal or deficient. The study would like to determine which, if any, of the vitamin/mineral levels are linked to differences in IQ.
2. A study is investigating the link between red wine intake and cholesterol level. Volunteers have been recruited and split into 3 groups depending on their weekly red wine intake. Cholesterol levels have been recorded for each volunteer. The study would like to determine if there is any difference in cholesterol levels between the groups.
3. A clinical trial is evaluating the efficacy of a new painkiller. Patients on the trial were given either the new drug or an existing painkilling drug. They were asked to record the level of pain they experienced. The trial would like to establish if the new drug was a more effective painkiller than the existing drug.
4. A study is investigating differences in physical development between ethnic groups. Volunteers from five different ethnic groups have been recruited. Height and weight data have been recorded from all volun-

teers. The study would like to determine if there are any differences in height and/or weight between the ethnic groups.

5. A team of biomedical engineers is evaluating a new robotic surgical technique. A patient cohort has been identified, half of the patients (randomly selected) underwent conventional surgery, and the other half underwent robotic surgery. The surgery time in minutes and the subsequent hospital stay in days were recorded for each patient. The team would like to know if there was any difference in surgery time and/or hospital stay between the patients who underwent the two types of surgery.

8.5 SUMMARY

If we are interested in performing multiple hypothesis tests on a single set of data, there is an increased chance of at least one type I error occurring. Bonferroni's correction is a simple adjustment that can maintain the chance of a type I error at less than the significance level. It works by dividing the critical significance level by the number of tests being performed.

ANOVA (analysis of variance) is a test that can be applied in cases where there are multiple groups of data, and we are interested in determining if their means are the same or not. It works by computing two different estimates of the population variance, one of which is sensitive to differences in mean between groups, and the other of which is not.

Multivariate data refers to having more than one variable for each "individual". Hotelling's T^2 test is a generalization of the Student's t-test to multivariate data.

Likewise, MANOVA (multivariate analysis of variance) is a generalization of the ANOVA test to multivariate data.

8.6 MULTIPLE AND MULTIVARIATE HYPOTHESIS TESTING USING MATLAB

There are built-in functions in the MATLAB Statistics and Machine Learning Toolbox for several of the tests that we have covered in this chapter. The sections below outline the basics of using these functions and also how MATLAB can be used to apply tests for which no built-in function exists. Please see the MATLAB documentation for more details.

8.6.1 Bonferroni's Correction

Although there are more sophisticated functions available, probably the most straightforward way to implement Bonferroni's correction in MATLAB is just to adjust the significance level of the hypothesis test yourself based on the number of tests. For example, the following code excerpt illustrates how this can be done for six tests and a significance level of 0.05:

```
nTests = 6;
sigLevel = 0.05;
... define data
[h,p] = ttest(sample1, sample2, 'alpha', sigLevel/nTests);
... apply other tests with same adjusted significance level
```

8.6.2 ANOVA

The MATLAB `anova1` function can be used for one way ANOVA tests using either balanced or unbalanced groups, as the following examples illustrate.

Balanced groups:

```
n = 10;
group1 = randn(n,1);
group2 = randn(n,1);
group3 = randn(n,1);
data = [group1, group2, group3];
p = anova1(data, {'G1','G2','G3'})
```

Unbalanced groups:

```
n1 = 10;
n2 = 15;
n3 = 20;
group1 = randn(n1,1);
group2 = randn(n2,1);
group3 = randn(n3,1);
data = [group1; group2; group3];
group_labels = [repmat('1', [n1 1]); repmat('2', [n2 1]); ...
                repmat('3', [n3 1])];
p = anova1(data, group_labels, {'G1','G2','G3'})
```

In both cases, group samples are drawn from the standard normal distribution (i.e. $\mu = 0$, $\sigma = 1$). In the balanced groups case, all groups have sample size 10, whereas in the unbalanced groups case, the group sample sizes are 10, 15, and 20.

The return argument `p` is the p-value of the test, so if this is less than the significance level, then the null hypothesis is rejected.

8.6.3 Hotelling's T^2 Test

There are no built-in functions in MATLAB for performing Hotelling's T^2 test. However, it is reasonably straightforward to implement the required operations as outlined in Section 8.3.1. The following code excerpts illustrate these operations for one- and two-sample paired data and for two-sample unpaired data cases, using variables randomly sampled from a normal distribution.

One-sample data:

```
n=10; % sample size
p=3; % number of variables
expected = [1 2 3]; % expected means

% generate data from normal distribution
var1 = randn(n,1) + expected(1);
var2 = randn(n,1) + expected(2);
var3 = randn(n,1) + expected(3);

% Hotelling's T2 test operations
X = [var1, var2, var3]; % sample matrix
C = cov(X);                 % covariance matrix
Xbar = mean(X,1);        % mean sample
T2 = n * (Xbar−expected) * inv(C) * (Xbar−expected)';
F = (n−p)/(p*(n−1)) * T2;
```

Two-sample paired data:

```
n=10; % sample size
p=3; % number of variables

% generate data from normal distribution
% data set A
varA1 = randn(n,1);
varA2 = randn(n,1);
varA3 = randn(n,1);
% data set B
varB1 = randn(n,1);
varB2 = randn(n,1);
varB3 = randn(n,1);

% Hotelling's T2 test operations
X = [varA1−varB1, varA2−varB2, varA3−varB3]; % sample matrix
expected = [0 0 0];
C = cov(X);                 % covariance matrix
Xbar = mean(X,1);        % mean sample
T2 = n * (Xbar−expected) * inv(C) * (Xbar−expected)';
F = (n−p)/(p*(n−1)) * T2;
```

Two-sample unpaired data:

```
nA=10; nB=15; % sample sizes
p=3; % number of variables

% generate data from normal distribution
% data set A
varA1 = randn(nA,1);
varA2 = randn(nA,1);
```

```
varA3 = randn(nA,1);
% data set B
varB1 = randn(nB,1);
varB2 = randn(nB,1);
varB3 = randn(nB,1);

% Hotelling's T2 test operations
XA = [varA1, varA2, varA3]; % sample matrix A
XB = [varB1, varB2, varB3]; % sample matrix B
CA = cov(XA);               % covariance matrix A
CB = cov(XB);               % covariance matrix B
C = ((nA-1)*CA + (nB-1)*CB)/(nA+nB-2);
XbarA = mean(XA,1);         % mean sample A
XbarB = mean(XB,1);         % mean sample B
T2 = (nA*nB)/(nA+nB)*(XbarA-XbarB)*inv(C)*(XbarA-XbarB)';
F = (nA+nB-p-1)/(p*(nA+nB-2)) * T2;
```

Alternatively, you can download an implementation of Hotelling's T^2 test from the Mathworks File Exchange (see Section 8.7).

8.6.4   MANOVA

The MATLAB `manova1` function can be used for one-way MANOVA tests for either balanced or unbalanced groups, as the following example illustrates:

```
nA=10; nB=15; nC=12; % sample sizes
p=3; % number of variables
alpha=0.05; % significance level

% Generate samples of size n=10 for groups A,B,C with
% p=3 variables, data drawn from standard normal distribution
groupA_var1 = randn(nA,1);
groupA_var2 = randn(nA,1);
groupA_var3 = randn(nA,1);
groupB_var1 = randn(nB,1);
groupB_var2 = randn(nB,1);
groupB_var3 = randn(nB,1);
groupC_var1 = randn(nC,1);
groupC_var2 = randn(nC,1);
groupC_var3 = randn(nC,1);

% prepare data for MATLAB function
data = [groupA_var1, groupA_var2 groupA_var3; ...
        groupB_var1, groupB_var2 groupB_var3; ...
        groupC_var1, groupC_var2 groupC_var3];
groups = [repmat('A', [nA 1]); repmat('B', [nB 1]); ...
          repmat('C', [nC 1])];

[d,p,stats] = manova1(data, groups, alpha)
```

In this example, all samples are drawn from the standard normal distribution (i.e. $\mu = 0$, $\sigma = 1$). The sample sizes of groups A, B, and C are 10, 15, and 12, although these can be set the same for the balanced groups case. A value for the return argument d that is greater than zero means that we can reject the null hypothesis that the group multivariate means are the same at the given significance level alpha.

8.7 FURTHER RESOURCES

- Although Bonferroni's correction is widely understood and applied, a number of alternatives do exist, which may provide more statistical power. For example, the Holm–Bonferroni method or the Šidák correction can also be used to control the *familywise error rate*:
  https://en.wikipedia.org/wiki/Holm-Bonferroni_method,
  https://en.wikipedia.org/wiki/Šidák_correction.
- There is a free online calculator for critical F values for the ANOVA and Hotelling's T^2 tests available at
  https://www.danielsoper.com/statcalc/calculator.aspx?id=4
- Tukey's HSD test is an alternative to the ANOVA test that provides more specific information; it also reveals which of the pairs of means was significantly different:
  https://en.wikipedia.org/wiki/Tukey's_range_test
- The Kruskal–Wallis test is a nonparametric alternative to the ANOVA test that does not require the assumption of normality:
  https://en.wikipedia.org/wiki/Kruskal-Wallis_one-way_analysis_of_variance
- In this book, we have described how to perform a one-way ANOVA test, which is applicable when there is a single factor under investigation. Two-way ANOVA tests can be used when there are two factors; see, for example, http://www.biostathandbook.com/twowayanova.html
- A MATLAB implementation for Hotelling's T^2 test can be downloaded from the Mathworks File Exchange:
  https://mathworks.com/matlabcentral/fileexchange/2844-hotellingt2
- Further details of the mathematics behind the MANOVA test can be found at
  http://online.sfsu.edu/efc/classes/biol710/manova/manovanewest.htm

8.8 EXERCISES

- Exercise 8.1

O8.A   In Activity 8.1, we introduced an example of using fMRI to test for differences in brain oxygenation level between rest and performing a task. The rest and task data for each of the five brain regions are available in the file "fmri.mat" from the book's web site. Use MATLAB to repeat the Student's t-tests with Bonferroni's correction.

■ **Exercise 8.2**

In Exercise 6.10 we introduced the *standardized uptake value* (SUV) as a measure of tumor activity in positron emission tomography (PET) imaging. A high SUV value indicates a metabolically active tumor.

O8.A

A new chemotherapy drug is being evaluated for treating cancer. The new drug is delivered in addition to standard chemotherapy drugs. A cohort of 100 cancer patients has been recruited and split into groups of 20. The first group (the *control*) received only the standard chemotherapy drugs. The next four groups all also received the new drug at varying doses. The researchers wish to know which, if any, of the four groups taking the new drug had lower tumor SUV values than the control group.

The SUV values are available in the file "suv_values.mat" from the book's web site. Write a MATLAB script to load in the data and answer the researchers' question. You can assume that all data are normally distributed with equal variance. Work to a 95% degree of confidence.   ■

■ **Exercise 8.3**

In Section 8.2.2, we introduced a case study on treatment of Alzheimer's disease patients. The MMSE score differences for the four treatment groups are available in the file "mmse_diffs.mat" from the book's web site. Use MATLAB to repeat the ANOVA test that we performed by hand in Section 8.2.2.   ■

O8.B

■ **Exercise 8.4**

In Activity 8.2, we introduced the example of determining if the mean peak ejection rate (PER) varied between heart failure patients in different NYHA classes. Use MATLAB to repeat the ANOVA test that you performed by hand in Activity 8.2. The data are available in the file "per_data.mat".   ■

O8.B

■ **Exercise 8.5**

In Section 8.3.1, we introduced a case study on the links between diet and depression. The data are available to you in the file "diet_data.mat" from the book's web site. Use MATLAB to repeat the Hotelling's T^2 test that we performed by hand in Section 8.3.1, that is, compute the covariance matrix, the T^2 value, and the F statistic using MATLAB commands.   ■

O8.C

■ **Exercise 8.6**

Now repeat the Hotelling's T^2 test that you performed in Activity 8.3. The original data are available in the file "blood_serum.mat". Use MATLAB to compute the covariance matrix, the T^2 value, and the F statistic and compare the latter to the critical F value.   ■

O8.C

■ Exercise 8.7

O8.C   A study is assessing the efficacy of a new treatment for respiratory dysfunction. Common indicators of respiratory function include:

■ Pulse oximetry (SpO2): the level of oxygen in the blood, measured as a percentage.
■ Forced vital capacity (FVC): the volume of the lungs measured from a full breath in to a full breath out, measured in cm^3.
■ Maximal inspiratory pressure (MIP): a test of the strength of the muscles used to breathe in, measured in cmH_2O.

A group of 30 patients suffering from respiratory dysfunction has been recruited onto the study. The three parameters listed were measured before and after treatment. In addition, a reference cohort of 20 healthy volunteers also had the same indicators measured. All data are available in the file "respiratory.mat" from the book's web site.

Assuming that all data are normally distributed and working to a 95% degree of confidence, answer the following questions:

1. Are the indicators of respiratory function significantly different between the healthy volunteers and the patients before treatment?
2. Are the indicators of respiratory function for the patients significantly different between the before and after treatment data?   ■

■ Exercise 8.8

O8.D   Consider the extension to the cognitive function example that we introduced in Section 8.3.2. Recall that we now have three variables recorded for each subject: the differences in scores for the Mini Mental State Examination (MMSE), the Alzheimer's Disease Assessment Scale (cognitive subscale, ADAS-cog), and the Severe Impairment Battery (SIB). We have these values for patients in each of four treatment groups: *none*, *mental stimulation*, *physical exercise*, and *drug*. Each group has 25 patients. These data are available in the file "alzheimers_multivariate.mat".

Use MATLAB to perform a one-way MANOVA test to determine, with 95% confidence, whether the means of the four groups of data are the same or not.   ■

FAMOUS STATISTICIAN: RONALD FISHER

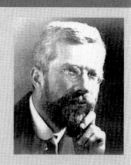

Ronald Fisher is one of the major figures in the history of statistics and is sometimes referred to as the "Father of Statistics". He was born in 1890 in East Finchley, London, and was the son of a successful London art dealer. However, soon after Ronald's birth, his father lost his fortune. His mother died when he was 14. Ronald was a brilliant mathematician and went on to study at Cambridge University.

Whilst at Cambridge, he developed an interest in the controversial field of "eugenics", which proposes the use of selective breeding to improve the genetic traits of the human race. Shortly before he graduated from Cambridge in 1912, his tutor informed him that, despite his enormous aptitude for scientific work and his mathematical potential, his disinclination to show calculations or to prove propositions rendered him unsuited for a career in applied mathematics, which required greater fortitude. His tutor gave him a "lukewarm" recommendation, stating that if Fisher "had stuck to the ropes he would have made a first-class mathematician, but he would not." Despite his tutor's reservations, Ronald Fisher went on to have an extremely distinguished career as a statistician. His contributions to the field include the theory of Analysis of Variance (ANOVA) and Fisher's exact test (a statistical significance test used in the analysis of contingency tables; see Chapter 2).

A defining theme of Ronald Fisher's life was his long running feud with another of the most significant figures in the history of statistics, Karl Pearson (see Chapter 1's Famous Statistician). In fact, the name "Fisher's exact test" was intended as an indirect criticism of Karl Pearson's chi-square test (see Chapter 6), which he considered to be inexact and which he intended to replace. Fisher died aged 72 in 1962 in Adelaide, Australia.

"Fisher was a genius who almost single-handedly created the foundations for modern statistical science"

Anders Hald

CHAPTER 9

Experimental Design and Sample Size Calculations

9.1 INTRODUCTION

The preceding chapters have introduced a variety of statistical techniques and tests. When applying these tests, it has generally been assumed that the experiment has already been carried out and the results gathered. The task was just to statistically analyze the data provided. In practice, an effective researcher will consider the method by which he will analyze their results right from the start of the experimental process. In the words of Ronald Fisher, the "Father of Statistics",

> "To consult the statistician after an experiment is finished is often merely to ask him to conduct a post mortem examination. He can perhaps say what the experiment died of."

This chapter will explore how, by taking care with experimental design, more accurate results, and less biased results can be gathered. This, in turn, will result in more powerful findings and fewer incorrect conclusions.

9.2 EXPERIMENTAL AND OBSERVATIONAL STUDIES

When gathering statistical data, there are two main ways in which studies can be designed, *experimental* and *observational* studies. These were briefly discussed

Statistics for Biomedical Engineers and Scientists. https://doi.org/10.1016/B978-0-08-102939-8.00018-9

in Section 2.2.4 in the context of plotting graphs and deciding which variable should go on which axis. In this chapter, the two types of study will be discussed in more detail, and new statistical notation introduced.

9.2.1 Observational Studies

In observational studies the researcher does not directly control the variables under investigation. An example would be an investigation into the risk of developing lung cancer for smokers and nonsmokers. We might choose to have two variables (smoker/nonsmoker and cancer/no cancer) and simply gather data for the two variables by using questionnaires or accessing existing health records. However, we could not control who gets cancer, and we would not control who smoked and who did not.[1]

Observational studies can be *forward-looking* (or *prospective*), in which a group (often called a *cohort*) of participants is selected and then followed over time. Alternatively, they can be *backward-looking* (or *retrospective*), where, for example, participants with a particular disease (plus matched controls) are enrolled onto the study, and then their past is investigated to determine factors that could have led to catching the disease.

A *prospective* study over a period of time (a *prospective longitudinal study*) is often called a *cohort study*. A *retrospective longitudinal study* is often called a *case control study*.

Observational studies are generally considered to be weaker than experimental studies in terms of statistical power, that is, observational studies will generally need more data to show the same effect. This is because it is harder to minimize errors when we have no control over the experimental environment.

9.2.2 Experimental Studies

In experimental studies the researcher is able to control many aspects of the environment in which the experiment takes place. They are able to alter the values of particular variables and then measure responses. By having control over the environment the researcher can try to minimize factors that could obscure the experimental results.

There are three main elements to an experimental study:

- *Experimental units.* These are the individual objects or subjects under investigation.
- *Treatments.* This refers to the procedures that are applied to each unit in the experimental study.

---

[1] At least, it would be unethical to do so!

■ *Responses*. This refers to the measurements by which the different treatments will be compared.

The aim of any experimental study is to clearly show the difference in *response* when different *treatments* are applied to the *experimental units* (assuming of course that the researchers' hypothesis is correct and a difference does in fact exist). Differences will be obscured by variations in the responses which are due to factors other than the treatments under investigation. Good experimental design will attempt to minimize these obscuring variations.

9.2.3 Showing Cause-and-Effect

In an experimental study, because the researcher has control over some of the variables, the study can be used to show a *cause-and-effect* relationship. However, observational studies can only show that there is a relationship between variables but cannot show cause-and-effect. That is because *confounding variables* may be present. A confounding variable is a variable related to the other variables under investigation in such a way that it makes it impossible to distinguish whether the effect is caused by one of the measured variables or the confounding variable. For example, a study was carried out relating gender to salary scales for nurses in a particular hospital. The study found that female nurses have higher mean salaries than male nurses. However, it was also found that female nurses have more years of experience. In this case, years of experience was a confounding variable. From the study we cannot tell whether the salary difference is due to gender discrimination or years of experience.

■ **Activity 9.1**

State whether each of the following scenarios is an observational or experimental study. Explain your answers.   *O9.A*

1. Blood pressure data have been recorded from two groups of volunteers. One of the groups was known to have an active lifestyle, and the other was known to have a sedentary lifestyle. The investigators would like to know if the average blood pressures of the two groups are significantly different.

2. To investigate the safe level of energy deposition in cardiac catheter ablation interventions, an experiment has been performed on animals in which the subjects underwent ablation using different levels of energy deposition. The survival or death of the subject was recorded, and this was used to divide the energy deposition data into two data sets. The investigators would like to know whether the distributions of the energy deposition values are different between the surviving and deceased groups of subjects.

■

9.3 RANDOM AND SYSTEMATIC ERROR (BIAS)

All measurements in the real world contain some amount of error. These errors can be split into two main types:

- *Random error.* These are errors that fluctuate randomly around a central value. Therefore, if many measurements are repeated, and a mean value calculated, then the errors would eventually cancel out. These errors have no observable pattern: they are random. They are the types of errors which statistical analysis is designed to deal with, and can be modeled by probability distributions (e.g. a Gaussian or t-distribution).
- *Systematic error* (or *bias*). These errors have a consistent pattern, which is not due to chance. For example, if a researcher measured distances with an ultrasound probe in a water bath (sound velocity in water = 1500 m/s) when the probe was calibrated for human tissue (sound velocity in human tissue = 1540 m/s), this would result in all of the distances measured being too large by a factor of 1540/1500. In other words, there would be a bias in the measurements. Systematic errors are difficult to detect. They are *not* picked up by statistical analysis and can often be the cause of incorrect experimental conclusions. Collecting more data will not help to minimize the effect of a systematic error: a biased sample is biased regardless of its size. However, because a bias is systematic and so repeatable, if the bias is known, then it can often be removed. Removal of bias is one of the main aims of good experimental design.

■ Activity 9.2

O9.A   For each of the examples below, explain the nature of the errors. Are they due to random error or is a systematic error or bias involved?

1. A study needs to regularly measure the heights of a group of children and compare them with those of a second cohort of children of the same age. The parents are instructed to always carry out the measurements first thing in the morning. The results show some variation, but the children are significantly taller than the second cohort.
2. To obtain a value for a patient's heart volume, ten cardiologists manually draw around the heart boundary in a magnetic resonance (MR) scan. The cardiologists are given detailed instructions on which features to draw around. The results differ slightly.
3. A student wants to know if it is quicker to travel by bicycle or train to get to a 9am lecture. They alternate every week between bicycle and train and record their travel times. There is variation in both sets of times, but more variation in the train travel times.

■

9.4 REDUCING RANDOM AND SYSTEMATIC ERRORS

9.4.1 Blocking (Matching) Test and Control Subjects

Researchers are often interested in demonstrating that their new experimental method (the *test*) is better than an established method (the *control*). To most clearly observe the effect of the new method, the test and control experiments should be carried out in as similar a fashion as is reasonably possible. The aim is to reduce random variation, so that the treatment effect can be observed.

If possible it is preferable to carry out a *within-subject* design, in which the same experimental unit acts as both test and control. For example, if a new drug was being tested, then this could be achieved by obtaining a control baseline measurement from an individual before administering the drug, and then afterward obtaining a test measurement from the same individual.

However, it is often not practical to use a within-subject design. For instance, suppose we were interested in investigating the long-term prognosis after undergoing (or not undergoing) a surgical procedure – it is not possible for a single individual to both have and not have the procedure. In these cases a *between-subjects* design, in which different subjects are compared, must be used. Because different subjects are compared, there will be variations due to the different individuals in the test and control groups. If possible, individuals in the test and control groups should be *matched* over as many variables as possible to reduce unwanted variations. To return to the surgical procedure example, we might try to match subjects according to variables such as age, gender, or aspects of their clinical history.

A *randomized block design* involves subjects being split into two groups (or blocks) such that the variation within the groups (according to the chosen matching variables) is less than the variation between the groups. Subjects within each block are then assigned randomly to one of the treatments (e.g. having the surgical procedure or not having it). A special case of the randomized block design is the *matched pairs design*, in which there are only two treatments and a one-to-one correspondence is established between pairs of subjects based on the matching variables (i.e. they are matched pairs). Subjects from each pair are then randomly assigned to one of the two treatments.

9.4.2 Blinding

Systematic errors can arise because either the participants or the researchers have particular knowledge about the experiment. Probably the best known example is the *placebo effect*, in which patients' symptoms can improve simply because they believe that they have received some treatment even though, in reality, they have been given a treatment of no therapeutic value (e.g. a sugar pill). What is less well known, but nevertheless well established, is that the behavior of researchers can alter in a similar way. For example, a researcher who knows that a participant has received a specific treatment may monitor the participant much more carefully than a participant who he/she knows has received no treatment. *Blinding* is a method to reduce the chance of these effects causing a bias. There are three levels of blinding:

1. *Single-blind.* The participant does not know if he/she is a member of the treatment or control group. This normally requires the control group to receive a placebo. Single-blinding can be easy to achieve in some types of experiments, for example, in drug trials the control group could receive sugar pills. However, it can be more difficult for other types of treatment. For example, in surgery there are ethical issues involved in patients having a placebo (or sham) operation.[2]
2. *Double-blind.* Neither the participant nor the researcher who delivers the treatment knows whether the participant is in the treatment or control group.
3. *Triple-blind.* Neither the participant, the researcher who delivers the treatment, nor the researcher who measures the response knows whether the participant is in the treatment or control group.

9.4.3 Multiple Measurement

In real-world experiments, there will be errors in response measurement. These may be due to the measurement device used or variations between how different researchers (or the same researcher) measure the response. These types of variation can all be investigated by taking multiple measurements. In particular, it is common to measure two specific types of variation:

- *Intraobserver variability* refers to variations in the measurements made by a single researcher. These may be due to the measurement device used or simply the researcher performing the measurement slightly differently each time. Assessing intraobserver variability requires the same researcher to make the same measurement multiple times.
- *Interobserver variability* refers to variations in the measurements made by different researchers. Assessing this requires a number of different researchers to make the same measurement.

These values can be useful indicators of the accuracy of the measured values and can be useful in detecting systematic errors. If the errors are random, then taking the average of multiple measurements can reduce the errors.

---

[2] But these are sometimes performed: http://en.wikipedia.org/wiki/Sham_surgery

9.4.4   Randomization

Researchers often want to infer that their results apply to a population (not just the experimental sample). To make such an inference, the sample taken must be a representative random sample from the population under study. This can be difficult to achieve. For example, if we are carrying out a day time landline telephone survey, then even if we randomly pick numbers from the telephone directory, we are limiting our sample participants to those who: 1) have a landline telephone, 2) are at home to answer the telephone during the day, 3) are not ex-directory, and 4) are willing to spend time participating in the survey. Care would need to be taken if the results from such a survey were used to make inferences about the general population. Similarly, in the biomedical field, when a new operation is tested, it may be the patient population who are not suitable for the standard procedure who are offered the new treatment. These could be higher-risk patients, which would lead to a negative bias, and it might be difficult to obtain suitable control cases.

Potential bias can often be reduced by using random selection, in particular:

- Random selection of participants (experimental units).
- Random allocation of participants to test or control groups.
- Random ordering of treatment or placebo (in a *within-subject* design).

■ Activity 9.3

Consider the following two case studies and then complete the tasks listed: *O9.B, O9.C*

1. You have developed a new hard wearing shoe sole material. You want to obtain evidence that it is better than the currently used material. You formulate a hypothesis: the new material will wear down 20% less than the current material.
2. You have designed a new drug, which can improve people's academic performance for 3 hours after it is taken. You want to show its effect to publish a paper. You have designed an IQ test. You formulate a hypothesis: the smart drug will make people perform 20% better in the IQ test.

Tasks:

a Write down a brief initial experimental design for each case study indicating how you would investigate the hypotheses. At this stage, consider the following questions only. What will your experimental units be? What will your treatment be? How will you measure response?
b Identify any potential systematic errors (biases) in your experiment.
c Identify any sources of random error in your experiment.

　　　　d Consider possible ways in which you could reduce the above sources
　　　　　of error. For instance, the techniques that we have discussed in this
　　　　　chapter have been: blocking (matching) test and control, blinding,
　　　　　multiple measurements, and randomization.
　　　　e Write down a final experimental design.

9.5　SAMPLE SIZE AND POWER CALCULATIONS

Typically, a researcher aims to show that a proposed treatment has a response
that is statistically significantly different from a known value or from the response of the current (control) treatment. To achieve this, they perform an
experiment and gather some data. How can they maximize their chance of
being able to find statistical significance using the data gathered?

Let us consider the case of testing a single sample against a known value.
Eq. (5.1) defined the test statistic for the one-sample t-test. This equation is
reproduced here for convenience:

$$t = \frac{\bar{x} - \mu}{s/\sqrt{n}}.$$

Recall that $\bar{x}$ is the test sample mean, μ is the value we are comparing against,
s is the standard deviation of the test sample, and n is the sample size. To
increase our chance of achieving statistical significance, the absolute value of t
must be as large as possible. So what do we have control of in this equation?

- $\bar{x} - \mu$ is the difference that we aim to demonstrate. We probably cannot
  make this value any larger as we have presumably already designed our
  new method so that its results x are as good as possible (i.e. as different
  from μ as possible).
- s is the sample standard deviation. By careful experimental design this
  can be made as small as possible, but variations will remain.
- n is the sample size. This is a parameter that we potentially have full control of. So long as there are no other constraints (e.g. financial or ethical),
  we could make n large enough to show a statistically significantly differ-
  ence for any $\|\bar{x} - \mu\| > 0$.

With this in mind, *sample size* calculations allow us to work out how large n
needs to be in order to be likely to achieve statistical significance at a given
significance level (e.g. 0.05 or 0.01). To perform a sample size calculation, we
must decide how high we want our chance of achieving significance to be. This
probability of success is known as the *power* of our experiment, and typical
values used are 0.8 or 0.9.

Alternatively, *power* calculations enable us to work out the probability of an experiment finding a significant difference (if it exists) given a sample size n for a specified significance level.

9.5.1 Illustration of a Power Calculation for a Single Sample *t*-test

Consider the following example. A new x-ray detector is being developed, which is predicted to be able to produce images with a mean signal-to-noise ratio (SNR) of 110 compared to a mean value of 100 for a standard detector. We can form the following hypotheses:

- *Null hypothesis*. The new x-ray detector has a mean SNR of 100.
- *Alternative hypothesis*: The new x-ray detector has a mean SNR that is significantly greater than 100.

We acquire 16 images with the new detector and measure the SNR for each one. Based on these data, we could apply a single sample *t*-test to test the hypotheses. A power calculation can be used to answer the question: *What is the probability that this experiment will be able to show a statistically significant difference at a given significance level?* To carry out this calculation, an estimate of the standard deviation of the values measured is required. This is usually obtained from prior data or from a small pilot study. In this case, let us assume that the standard deviation of the sample is 20.

Fig. 9.1 shows the estimated probability distribution of the mean SNR measured by the experiment *assuming that the null hypothesis is true*. The critical value (for a 1-tailed test, at 0.05 significance) at which the null hypothesis would be rejected is 108.8. Therefore, if the mean SNR value from the experiment is 108.8 or larger, then the experiment will show a statistically significant difference.

Now if the predicted value of SNR = 110 for the new x-ray detector is correct, what is the probability that the experiment will result in a mean SNR of greater than 108.8? To answer this question, we consider an additional probability distribution as shown in Fig. 9.2. This is the distribution of mean SNR values that would result from the experiment *assuming that the predicted SNR of 110 is correct*. The newly shaded area represents the probability that the experiment will produce a mean SNR that is greater than 108.8. In this example, the magenta shaded area represents 60% of the total area of the distribution, and so in statistical notation, we would write that the experiment has a statistical *power* of 60%.

In most situations, this would be considered to be an *underpowered* experiment. Typical values of power used are 80% or 90%. In the next section, we illustrate how to determine the sample size required to reach this power.

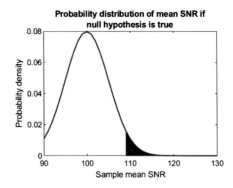

FIGURE 9.1
Estimated probability distribution of the mean SNR assuming that the null hypothesis is true (i.e. our new x-ray detector mean SNR = 100). The graph shows a t-distribution for 15 degrees of freedom centered at 100 with a standard deviation of $20/\sqrt{16} = 5$. The shaded area shows 5% of the total area for a 1-tailed critical value at 0.05 significance. The critical value is 108.8.

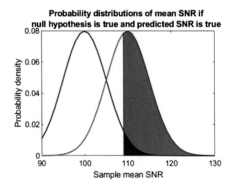

FIGURE 9.2
Estimated probability distributions of the means assuming that the null hypothesis is true (SNR = 100, blue curve) and assuming that our predicted value is true (SNR = 110, magenta curve). 60% of the area under the predicted mean distribution curve has an SNR greater than the 0.05 significance critical value of 108.8.

9.5.2 Illustration of a Sample Size Calculation

If the calculations carried out in the previous section were repeated for a range of different sample sizes n, then, for each n, the experiment would have a different power. Fig. 9.3 shows these powers plotted against n. The graph shows that a sample size of $n = 26$ is required to reach 80% power, and $n = 36$ is required to reach 90% power in this experiment. Notice also the way in which the graph curves: there are diminishing returns for each experimental unit that is added. This is because the standard error decreases in proportion to $\sqrt{n}$. Fig. 9.4 shows how the distributions change as n is increased from 12 up to 36.

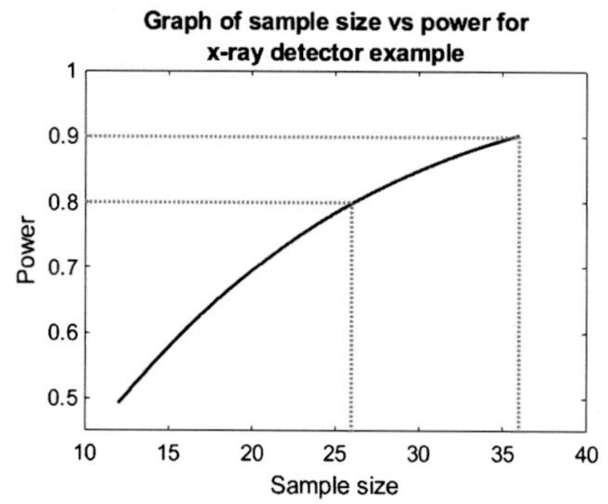

FIGURE 9.3
Graph of estimated power against sample size for the x-ray detector case study.

9.6 SUMMARY

There are many reasons, not least financial and ethical considerations, as to why experiments should use a sufficient but minimal amount of data to answer a research question. Good experimental design can enable the amount of data required to be reduced and can help to remove bias that could result in misleading experimental results. Carrying out power and sample size calculations helps to prevent experiments from being carried out, which would be very unlikely to reveal a true significant difference and also prevents the gathering of unnecessarily large data sets.

When designing experiments, a researcher must be very mindful of possible bias, which can be reduced using randomization, matched controls, and blinding techniques. A good experimental design should make analysis easier. As we have seen in this book so far there are many different statistical tests. A test can usually be found to fit most data sets. However, the more powerful tests generally perform better if the data are *balanced*; in other words, we have equal numbers of experimental units in each treatment block (e.g. equal numbers of test and control subjects).

The available tests differ greatly in their assumptions: for example, parametric versus nonparametric, 1-tailed versus 2-tailed, require paired data, require equal-sized samples, and so on. Essentially, the more assumptions a test requires, the more powerful it is likely to be, and the less data will be needed to show an effect. However, the more assumptions a test requires, the more difficult it can be to design an experiment producing data that fit with these assumptions. Often, small changes in experimental design and method can produce better data and enable the use of more powerful statistical tests.

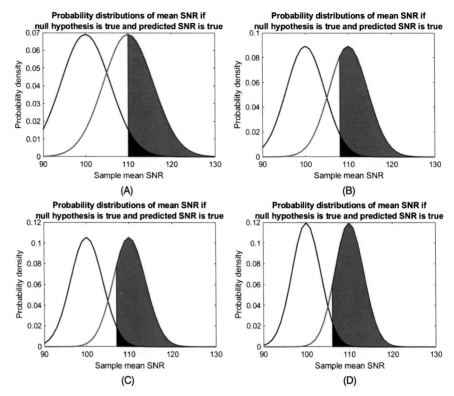

FIGURE 9.4

Graphs showing how probability distributions of the mean change as n is increased: (A) $n = 12$, (B) $n = 20$, (C) $n = 28$, and (D) $n = 36$. The blue shaded areas show the critical t-test values assuming that the null hypothesis is true. The magenta curves show the distributions of mean values assuming that the predicted SNR of 110 is true. The magenta shaded areas show the proportion of mean SNR values that would result in rejection of the null hypothesis. As n increases, the standard deviation decreases and the distributions become more separated, resulting in an increase in statistical power for the experiments for greater n.

9.7 POWER AND SAMPLE SIZE CALCULATIONS USING MATLAB

In MATLAB, there is a built-in function for power and sample size calculations for selected simple statistical tests.

9.7.1 Sample Size Calculations

```
n = sampsizepwr(testtype,p0,p1,power,  [])
```

Computes the sample size n for an experiment of the given testtype (e.g. a value of 't' can be used for a t-test). The argument p0 should be a vector containing the sample mean and standard deviation assuming that the null hypothesis is true, p1 is the predicted mean value, and power is the required power.

For example, to compute the required sample size to obtain a power of 90% in the x-ray detector experiment described in Section 9.5.1, we would use the following code:

```
n=sampsizepwr('t', [100 20], 110, 0.9, [], 'tail', 'right')
```

Note that we add two additional arguments to indicate that the *t*-test should be a right-tailed test, in a similar way to the ttest function introduced in Chapter 5.

9.7.2 Power Calculations

```
power = sampsizepwr(testtype,p0,p1,[],n
```

Computes the power for an experiment of the given testtype. The argument p0 should be a vector containing the sample mean and standard deviation assuming that the null hypothesis is true, p1 is the predicted mean value, and n is the sample size.

For example, to obtain the power for the x-ray detector experiment described in Section 9.5.1, we would use the following code.

```
power=sampsizepwr('t', [100 20], 110, [], 16, ...
                  'tail', 'right')
```

See the MATLAB documentation for the sampsizepwr function for details of which tests are implemented.

9.8 FURTHER RESOURCES

- A range of online sample size and power calculators is available at http://powerandsamplesize.com/
- More examples on the use of sampsizepwr can be found at http://mathworks.com/help/stats/examples/selecting-a-sample-size.html

9.9 EXERCISES

Perform the following tasks, either by hand or using MATLAB as indicated.

■ Exercise 9.1

A team of biomedical engineers has developed a new design for a "blade" prosthetic limb, for use by amputee athletes. They believe that their new design will enable athletes to run faster than they would using current designs, but would like to verify this hypothesis using statistical analysis.   *O9.A, O9.B, O9.C*

Design an experiment (by hand) to help the engineers to verify their hypothesis. In your description, you should address the following points:

- What type of study will be performed?
- What type of data will be gathered?
- How will the data be gathered?
- What possible sources of error are there and what will you do to minimize them?
- How will the data be statistically analyzed?

■ Exercise 9.2

O9.A, O9.C

A manufacturer of wooden panels prides itself on accurately producing goods to customers' specifications. Recently it has been receiving complaints that its panels have been 1 mm too small. The manufacturer is concerned that their machine might be out of calibration. To check this, the manufacturer produces ten 1 m long panels. The manufacturers have two measuring devices:

- A wooden ruler, which is difficult to read and only has markings every cm. The measurement standard deviation of this ruler is 3 mm.
- A brass ruler, which is much easier to read with markings every 0.5 mm. The measurement standard deviation of this ruler is 0.3 mm.

To increase the accuracy of their measurements, the manufacturers ask each of their 10 employees to measure each panel with each ruler, resulting in 100 length measurements in cm for each ruler. These are available to you in the data files "wooden_ruler.mat" and "brass_ruler.mat". The measurements are carried out on a very cold day. Use MATLAB to carry out single-sample t-tests against an expected mean of 100 cm using both sets of ruler data and decide whether you think the manufacturers need to recalibrate their machine.

■ Exercise 9.3

O9.E

Use MATLAB to verify the result obtained in Section 9.5.1, which calculated a power of 60% for a null hypothesis mean of 100, a predicted mean of 110, a standard deviation of 20, a significance level of 0.05, and a sample size $n = 16$.

■ Exercise 9.4

O9.E

Use MATLAB to verify the result obtained in Section 9.5.2, which calculated a sample size $n = 36$ for a null hypothesis mean of 100, a predicted mean of 110, a standard deviation of 20, a significance level of 0.05, and a power of 90%.

■ **Exercise 9.5**

You have designed a new guidance system for minimally invasive endovascular surgery, which you believe will greatly reduce x-ray exposure. Current x-ray exposure during these operations is $1200\,Gy\cdot cm^2$. You estimate that your new guidance system should be able to reduce this to $1000\,Gy\cdot cm^2$. From a small pilot study you estimate the standard deviation of your results to be $500\,Gy\cdot cm^2$. Use MATLAB to determine how many patients you would need to include in your experiment to test your new system using a significance level of 0.05 and a power of 90%.   ■

O9.E

■ **Exercise 9.6**

A colleague asks for your help. They are carrying out an experiment on a new drug to reduce blood pressure, which is being tested on mice. The drug is expected to reduce mean blood pressure from 110 to 100 mmHg. The estimated standard deviation of the blood pressure measurements is 10 mmHg. Your colleague is proposing to carry out an experiment with 20 mice but is concerned about using more animals than necessary. Use MATLAB to calculate the power of the experiment and advise your colleague.   ■

O9.E

■ **Exercise 9.7**

Carry out a Monte Carlo simulation to verify the result obtained in Section 9.5.1, which calculated a power of 60% for a null hypothesis mean of 100, a predicted mean of 110, a standard deviation of 20, a significance level of 0.05, and a sample size $n = 16$. Use the MATLAB `randn` function to produce sets of random data, which will then need to be shifted and scaled to produce the correctly simulated data sets. Test each of these data sets against the null hypothesis mean using the `ttest` function. The power will be the percentage of successful tests.   ■

O9.E

FAMOUS STATISTICIAN: GERTRUDE MARY COX

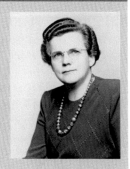

Gertrude Mary Cox was one of the leading figures in the field of experimental design. She was born in Dayton, Iowa, in 1900. After graduating from high school, she started studying to become a deaconess in the Methodist church. However, in 1925, she abandoned this plan and chose instead to study mathematics and statistics at Iowa State College. She graduated with a Batchelor's degree in 1929 and a Master's degree in 1931. In 1933, she got a job running the newly created Statistical Laboratory at Iowa State College.

In 1940, North Carolina State College was looking for a new Professor of Statistics. They contacted Gertrude's manager at Iowa, George Snedecor. He drew up a list of potentially suitable candidates (who were all men) and at the last minute showed it to Gertrude and asked her opinion. She is reported to have said "Why didn't you put my name on the list?" As a result, her name was added as a footnote to Snedecor's list with the comment "Of course if you would consider a woman for this position I would recommend Gertrude Cox of my staff". Gertrude got the job and became the first female Professor in the history of North Carolina State College.

In 1950, together with her colleague, William Cochrane, Gertrude published a seminal book in the history of statistics, entitled "Experimental Design". In it she and Cochrane wrote about factors such as the importance of good experimental design, the role of randomization in a good design, and sample size calculations. The book was hugely influential and became the major reference work for applied statisticians for many years.

In 1976, Gertrude found that she had leukemia. She fought bravely against her illness and remained upbeat until the end, referring to herself as "the experimental unit" whilst under treatment. She eventually succumbed to her illness and died in 1978 in Durham, North Carolina.

"She was a good person to know, both personally and professionally. She regarded her staff and their children very much as her family, and had their interests very much at heart."

Frank Yates

CHAPTER 10

Statistical Shape Models

LEARNING OBJECTIVES

At the end of this chapter, you should be able to:

O10.A *Describe what is meant by a statistical shape model (SSM)*
O10.B *Explain how SSMs make use of dimensionality reduction to estimate the variation of a population from a sample*
O10.C *Implement a simple landmark-based SSM in MATLAB*
O10.D *Give some examples of the use of SSMs in biomedical engineering*

10.1 INTRODUCTION

This chapter introduces the concept of *statistical shape modeling*. Statistical shape modeling is a technique that has been widely applied in the field of biomedical engineering since its proposal in the 1990s [9]. The content of this chapter might, at first, seem to be quite distinct from the concepts presented so far in this book. However, in effect, statistical shape models are strongly linked to the idea of *inferential statistics*. Just as with the techniques discussed in Chapters 4–8, statistical shape models are used to *infer* something about the population based on a sample drawn from it. Rather than just trying to infer some knowledge of a measure of *central tendency* (e.g. mean, median), they infer knowledge of likely *shapes* in a population of such shapes based on a sample drawn from it.

Statistical shape models (SSMs) have also been referred to as active shape models (ASMs) and point distribution models (PDMs) in the research literature. The meanings of these terms are very similar, but this text uses the term SSM throughout. This chapter begins by introducing the concept of statistical shape modeling and continues through the underlying theory and a review of some biomedical applications. At the end of the chapter, there is a guided exercise in which the reader can implement a simple SSM using MATLAB.

217

Statistics for Biomedical Engineers and Scientists. https://doi.org/10.1016/B978-0-08-102939-8.00019-0

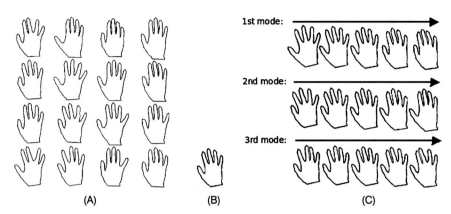

FIGURE 10.1

An illustration of a simple statistical shape model (SSM) reproduced from [9]. (A) A sample of the population of images of different hand shapes used to form the SSM. (B) The mean hand shape. (C) An illustration of the first three *modes of variation* of the resulting SSM: the first mode represents a general spreading of the fingers, the second mode is a separation of thumb and fingers, and the third mode is a separation of the index and middle fingers. The first mode of variation contains the largest amount of variation from the mean, followed by the second mode of variation, and so on.

10.2 SSMS AND DIMENSIONALITY REDUCTION

The basic idea of SSMs is to use a sample of shapes from a population to estimate not only the mean shape but also the statistical *modes of variation* of the population of such shapes. The term *modes of variation* refers to the dominant patterns of variation, and the idea is that any "realistic" example of what the population represents can be formed from the mean and a combination of a small number of these modes. For example, consider Fig. 10.1. Here, the sample data (Fig. 10.1A) are of the population of images of different hand outlines. The modes of variation (Fig. 10.1C) express how these images typically vary away from the mean hand shape (Fig. 10.1B). In this case the modes of variation involve different relative movements of the fingers and thumb. Any realistic hand shape can be expressed as a combination of these three modes of variation, that is, the three modes of variation are combined to *transform* the mean hand shape. There are obviously many possible transformations that are completely unrealistic (e.g. the index finger detaching itself from the hand), and so these will never be found in the population or any sample taken from it. Therefore these types of transformation will not be represented by the modes of variation. We can consider the modes of variation as a subset of all possible transformations that can be applied to a hand, with the subset representing only those that are likely to occur in real life. Clearly, the types of variation that will be captured by these modes will depend upon the variation that was present in the original sample, so to accurately estimate the population modes of variation, it is necessary to take a reasonable and representative sample for forming the SSM.

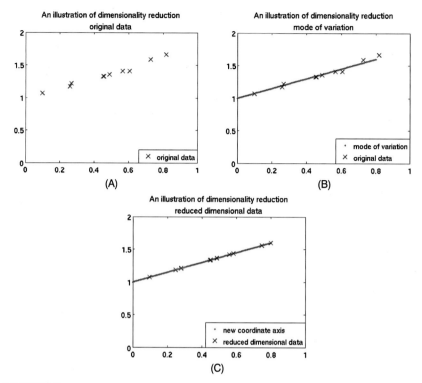

FIGURE 10.2

A simple illustration of the concept of *dimensionality reduction*. The plot in (A) shows a number of 2-D points. Two numbers (the x and y coordinates) are required to store each point, that is, the *dimensionality* of the data is 2. In (B) the dominant *mode of variation* of this data is shown. This illustrates that the 2-D points can be approximated by 1-D values. A single number for each point indicating how far it is along the solid line is sufficient to represent the same data, but with a reduced dimensionality of 1. These new data are shown in (C). We can think of this as defining a new, lower-dimensional, coordinate system, embedded in the original coordinate system. Note that this dimensionality reduction is, in this case, only an *approximation*: there will be some residual errors because not all points lie exactly on the solid line. The aim of dimensionality reduction techniques is typically to determine an estimate of the new coordinate system that minimizes these residual errors.

SSMs make use of a class of techniques known as *dimensionality reduction* techniques. Fig. 10.2 illustrates the concept of dimensionality reduction with a simple example. In this example, we can see how a set of 2-D points can be expressed as a set of 1-D points (i.e. scalar values), whilst still preserving most of the information in the original data. In other words, the *dimensionality* of the data has been reduced from 2 to 1. It is common, as in this example, that the dimensionality-reduced data are only an *approximation* to the original data. Note also that the solid line is a 2-D vector in the original coordinate system. Generally, each dimension of the lower-dimensional coordinate system is expressed as a vector in the higher-dimensional space.

So how do SSMs make use of dimensionality reduction to extract patterns of variation in data? Returning to the hands example, we can consider in detail the steps involved:

- First, each of the sample hands must be parameterized in some way, that is, reduced to a series of numbers. In this case the numbers represent the x and y coordinates of a number of points on each hand. These numbers must be *corresponding*, that is, they must represent the same anatomical location on different hands. So, for example, the first two numbers might represent the x and y coordinates of the tip of the index finger.

- Next, these parameterized shapes are plotted as points in a high-dimensional coordinate system. For example, suppose that we have 100 corresponding points on each hand. This means that our parameterization of each hand consists of 200 numbers. So each hand can be represented as a single point in a 200-dimensional coordinate system.

- Finally, dimensionality reduction is performed on the 200-dimensional points. The number of dimensions chosen for the lower-dimensional space can vary and is normally chosen with some domain knowledge. In the hand example, three dimensions were selected, meaning that new hand examples can be produced by specifying only three numbers, as opposed to the 200 in the original coordinate system. Note, however, that the hands produced in this way will still consist of 100 points, but the positions of these points will be generated from the three input numbers. As stated before, the axes of the lower-dimensional coordinate system are actually vectors in the high-dimensional coordinate system, so each vector represents a particular set of linear translations applied to the hand points (the translations for each point will be different). How this is exactly done is explained further in the next section.

10.3 FORMING AN SSM

In the following sections, we explain in more detail each of the steps involved in forming an SSM from a sample of shapes.

10.3.1 Parameterize the Shape

Starting with a sample of shapes, to estimate the modes of variation for these shapes, they must be represented in some way, for example, as digital images, sets of boundary points, and so on. The first stage of statistical shape modeling is to parameterize each shape in some way to form a vector of numbers, the *shape vector*. A common parameterization is to represent each shape by a set of landmark points, typically positioned on the boundaries of the shapes.

These landmarks can be located manually, automatically, or semiautomatically. However, one important feature of the point sequences is that there are exactly the same number of points defined for each shape and that they are *corresponding* points.

Now that each shape is represented by a sequence of points (most commonly in 2-D); the coordinates of the points can be concatenated into a single shape vector for each sample shape. Formally, for shape vector i consisting of K 2-D points $(x_{i,1}, y_{i,1}), \ldots, (x_{i,K}, y_{i,K})$, the shape vector $\mathbf{s}_i$ is

$$\mathbf{s}_i = \left[x_{i,1}, y_{i,1}, \ldots x_{i,K}, y_{i,K}\right]^T, \ 1 \le i \le n, \tag{10.1}$$

where n is the number of sample shapes.

10.3.2 Align the Centroids

It is often desirable to perform some type of *alignment* on the shape vectors before proceeding to form the SSM. For example, returning to the hands example shown in Fig. 10.1, suppose that the outlines were not positioned in the centers of the images. This would mean that the landmark coordinates would vary not just with the shape variation, but also with the position of the hand as a whole. This would cause an extra variation in the values of the shape vectors that would be extracted as a mode of variation by the SSM. If this is not desirable, then it is necessary to perform some alignment of the sample shapes to correct for this.

The simplest, and one of the most common, types of alignment is to align the *centroids* of all shapes. The *centroid* of a set of points is the mean point position, that is, the sum of all point coordinates divided by the number of points. By aligning the centroids of all sample shapes any *translational* differences between them are removed. Therefore, the shape vectors $\mathbf{s}_i$ can be redefined as follows:

$$\mathbf{s}_i = \left[x_{i,1} - \bar{x}_i, y_{i,1} - \bar{y}_i, \ldots x_{i,K} - \bar{x}_i, y_{i,K} - \bar{y}_i\right]^T, \ 1 \le i \le n, \tag{10.2}$$

where $(\bar{x}_i, \bar{y}_i)$ is the centroid of point sequence i, that is,

$$\bar{x}_i = \tfrac{1}{K} \sum_{k=1}^{K} x_{i,k}, \tag{10.3}$$

$$\bar{y}_i = \tfrac{1}{K} \sum_{k=1}^{K} y_{i,k}. \tag{10.4}$$

10.3.3 Compute the Mean Shape Vector

Once all of the sample shapes are aligned, the next stage is to compute the average shape. This is done by determining the *mean* shape vector of all n sample shapes,

$$\bar{\mathbf{s}} = \frac{1}{n} \sum_{i=1}^{n} \mathbf{s}_i. \tag{10.5}$$

This mean shape vector forms a part of the result of the SSM: all modes of variation will be expressed as variations from this mean.

10.3.4 Compute the Covariance Matrix

A key feature of SSMs is that they can determine and represent the modes of variation of data in a sample. In this case the data are sample shape vectors. Usually, the numbers in shape vectors will not vary independently – some numbers will change at the same time as certain other numbers. That is, there will be some nonzero *covariance* between the values of some of the elements of the shape vector. For example, in the hand example, points on the same finger will generally have similar movements. The *covariance matrix* introduced in Section 2.3.2 can be used to express these relationships between different vector elements. We compute the covariance matrix C as follows:

$$C = \frac{1}{n-1} \sum_{i=1}^{n} (\mathbf{s}_i - \bar{\mathbf{s}})(\mathbf{s}_i - \bar{\mathbf{s}})^T. \tag{10.6}$$

This equation is simply Eq. (2.3) reproduced using the notation of the shape vectors used in this chapter. Notice that the mean shape vector is subtracted from each sample shape vector to form the covariance matrix. Therefore, the matrix expresses the covariance away from this mean. The different elements of the covariance matrix indicate the covariances between the different elements of the shape vectors. For example, the element in row 1, column 3 of the matrix is the covariance between the 1st and 3rd elements of the shape vectors.

10.3.5 Compute the Eigenvectors and Eigenvalues

The final stage of building the SSM is to compute the *eigenvectors* and *eigenvalues* of the covariance matrix.

■ **Definition**
For an $M \times M$ matrix C, its eigenvectors $\mathbf{v}_1, \ldots, \mathbf{v}_M$ and (scalar) eigenvalues $\lambda_1, \ldots, \lambda_M$ are such that

$$C\mathbf{v}_m = \lambda_m \mathbf{v}_m$$

for all $1 \leq m \leq M$. ■

An important property of the eigenvectors and eigenvalues of a covariance matrix is that the eigenvectors represent the *principal components* of the variation of the data (e.g. the solid line in Fig. 10.2), and the eigenvalues represent the variance of the data along each eigenvector. Therefore, SSMs use the eigenvectors of the covariance matrix to allow dimensionality reduction to be performed.[1]

Formally, the eigenvectors $\mathbf{v}_m$ and eigenvalues λ_m of C are computed. The eigenvectors are all K-dimensional vectors (K is the number of elements in a shape vector), specifying a linear change to each number in the shape parameterization. Only eigenvectors with nonzero eigenvalues actually represent any variation in the data. The number of nonzero eigenvalues will be less than or equal to the sample size minus 1.

10.4 PRODUCING NEW SHAPES FROM AN SSM

The mean shape vector and the eigenvectors/eigenvalues together represent the SSM. This information can be used to generate new "realistic" examples of the population. To generate such a new example, a vector of *weights* must be specified, one weight for each eigenvector. These weights determine the relative contributions of the different modes of variation.

It is common to use a limited number of eigenvectors that are representative of the most significant variation in the data. For example, in the hands example only three eigenvectors (those that have the largest corresponding eigenvalues) were used, even though the covariance matrix had more than three nonzero eigenvalues. Typically, the number of eigenvectors is selected to ensure that the resulting SSM can account for a large percentage (e.g. 95%) of the total variation in the data.

Suppose that, based upon this criterion, the first c of M modes are selected. A new example of a shape vector $\hat{\mathbf{s}}$ can be produced as follows:

$$\hat{\mathbf{s}} = \bar{\mathbf{s}} + \sum_{m=1}^{c} b_m \mathbf{v}_m, \tag{10.7}$$

where $\bar{\mathbf{s}}$ is the mean shape, b_m represents the weight for mode m, and $\mathbf{v}_m$ is the corresponding eigenvector. In other words, a new shape vector is formed by adding a weighted sum of all eigenvectors to the mean shape vector.

It is common to allow the weights to vary only between prescribed limits. To allow them to take any value would result in unrealistic shapes. Since the eigenvalues represent the variance of the data along the eigenvectors, these can be used to limit the range of values for the weights. A common approach is to allow the weights to take any value in the range $-3\sqrt{\lambda_m} \leq b_m \leq +3\sqrt{\lambda_m}$, that is, plus or minus 3 standard deviations, in which case the SSM should capture more than 99% of the variation along each axis of the new lower-

---

[1]This technique is known as *principal component analysis* and was developed in 1901 by Karl Pearson; see the Famous Statistician for Chapter 1.

dimensional coordinate system (assuming the data are normally distributed; see Section 4.4.1).

10.5 BIOMEDICAL APPLICATIONS OF SSMS

SSMs have been used for a wide range of applications in biomedical engineering. In the original paper on SSMs [9] the proposed application was *segmentation*, or determining the outline of certain objects. In biomedical engineering, segmentation of organs or tumors can be very useful, for example, for visualization, surgical planning and guidance, or monitoring disease progression. In Chapter 3 (Exercise 3.3–Exercise 3.5) a clinical motivation for a basic segmentation tool was introduced with regard to hip prostheses. SSMs can be used to aid in segmentation of objects from images by varying the values of the weights, b_m, until the produced outline matches the object in the image. In this way the resulting segmentation will be limited to realistic examples of the object in question. For example, SSMs have been applied to segment the heart [10], as shown in Fig. 10.3. There are many other examples of the use of SSMs for segmenting different organs from medical images, and a good review can be found in [11].

Another application of SSMs in biomedical engineering is in analyzing the *motion* of organs. Organs in the thorax/abdomen move in a roughly repeatable way as we breathe. This motion can cause problems when acquiring medical images such as magnetic resonance (MR) scans: the motion of the organs causes artefacts in the images. Also, motion causes problems when using medical images to guide surgery since the real patient's organs will move whilst the organs in the images will not. SSMs have been used as a tool for parameterizing models of such motion with a view to overcoming these problems [13].

One more biomedical example of the use of SSMs is in *cardiac motion analysis*. Irregularities or changes in the motion of the heart as it beats can be indicative of the presence of some types of heart disease. By forming an SSM of the motion of the heart beat the resulting modes of variation can be analyzed and used to diagnose certain conditions [14]. This information can be useful for patient selection and planning of treatment.

■ Activity 10.1

O10.A, O10.B   A biomedical engineering company is trying to produce lower limb prosthetics for use in crisis situations. Under normal circumstances, these would be bespoke made for each individual, but they want to premanufacture a range of prosthetics for off-the-shelf use. How could they utilize statistical shape modeling to help in their manufacturing process?   ■

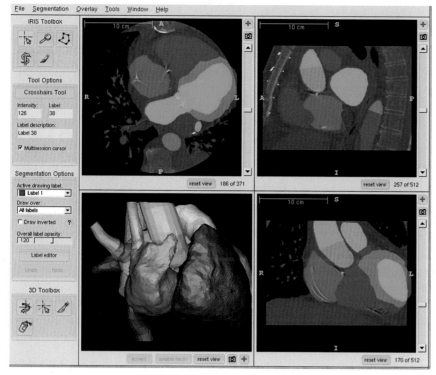

FIGURE 10.3

SSM-based whole heart segmentation from a computed tomography (CT) image [10], visualized using the ITK-SNAP software package [12] (http://www.itksnap.org). Top left, top right, bottom right panels: three orthogonal slices through the CT volume. Bottom left panel: surface rendering of segmentation. The four chambers and major vessels of the heart are rendered in different colors.

10.6 SUMMARY

Dimensionality reduction refers to the process of taking some very complex (i.e. high-dimensional) data and approximating it by some much simpler (i.e. lower-dimensional) data. SSMs are a common way of performing dimensionality reduction. They work by first parameterizing the complex data in some way to form a set of data vectors, then aligning the centroids of each vector, computing the mean data vector, and finally finding the eigenvalues and eigenvectors of the covariance matrix of the aligned vectors. The SSM is defined by the mean data vector and the eigenvectors/eigenvalues.

SSMs try to infer knowledge of likely shapes in a population based upon a sample drawn from it. They are a useful way of analyzing/describing the statistics of variation amongst a set of data and have found application in a range of different areas of biomedical engineering.

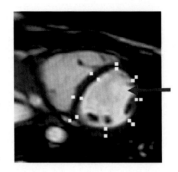

FIGURE 10.4
A 2D MR image of the left ventricle of the heart with boundary points indicated. The red arrow shows the left ventricle.

10.7   STATISTICAL SHAPE MODELING USING MATLAB

In the guided exercise in Section 10.9, you will construct a simple point-based SSM using MATLAB. Most of the MATLAB functionality required to form SSMs is based on common core functions, but the following specific function may be useful to you.

```
[v, d] = eig(c)
```

Determines the eigenvalues d and eigenvectors v of a covariance matrix c.

10.8   FURTHER RESOURCES

■ The original paper on SSMs by Cootes et al. [9] is quite accessible and worth reading. Although only published as recently as 1995, it has proved hugely influential in the field of biomedical engineering.
■ For a good review of applications of SSMs in medical image segmentation, see the paper by Heimann and Meinzer [11].

10.9   EXERCISES

In these exercises, you will use MATLAB to implement a simple SSM of the shape of the left ventricle of the heart. The data for the SSM have already been parameterized from a set of 2D magnetic resonance (MR) images of the left ventricle acquired from 20 different subjects: the parameterization consists of the x and y coordinates of a sequence of points on the inner and outer boundaries of the left ventricular myocardium. An example of such an image with the boundary points indicated is shown in Fig. 10.4.

■ **Exercise 10.1**

On the book's web site, for this chapter, you will find some MATLAB *m*-files   *O10.C*
that can be used to implement the SSM of the left ventricle data. However,
important parts of the code have been omitted. In this exercise, you will
implement these missing parts. The provided files include the following:

- ■ "main.m". This is the main script *m*-file that you should run. It loads
  the parameterized shape data into the workspace and calls the following functions.
- ■ "align_centroids.m'. The purpose of this function is to shift all 20 input shapes so that their centroids are at (0, 0). *This function is currently
  empty, and your task is to write this code.*
- ■ "create_ssm.m". The purpose of this function is to form the SSM from
  the aligned input shapes. This process consists of computing the mean
  shape vector, determining the covariance matrix and its eigenvectors
  and eigenvalues, and extracting the four eigenvectors with the largest
  eigenvalues. *This function is currently empty, and your task is to write this
  code.*
- ■ "vis_ssm.m". This is the function that sets up the user interface and
  allows visualization and interaction with the SSM. *This function is provided for you – you should not modify this file.*
- ■ "compute_coords_from_ssm.m". This function is used by "vis_ssm.m"
  to compute a shape vector from the SSM based on a set of weights for
  the modes of variation. *This function is provided for you – you should not
  modify this file.*

So, to summarize, your task is to write the code to complete the files
"align_centroids.m" and "create_ssm.m". Once complete, you should be able
to run the "main.m" script and visualize and interact with the SSM of the left
ventricle.   ■

■ **Exercise 10.2**

Try creating and visualizing the SSM without the centroid alignment step.   *O10.C*
What is the difference? Why?

*(Hint: In the MATLAB file "vis_ssm.m", you will need to change the axis limit
command to* `axis([30 120 30 120])` *to enable this visualization.)*   ■

■ **Exercise 10.3**

Try creating and visualizing the SSM using fewer data sets, that is, not all 20   *O10.C*
data sets. Can you notice any difference in the resulting SSM? If so, why?   ■

FAMOUS STATISTICIANS: JERZY NEYMAN AND GEORGE DANTZIG

For this chapter, we have two Famous Statisticians, George Dantzig and Jerzy Neyman. The reason they are included together is because their lives and works were strongly interlinked.

Neyman was a Polish–American mathematician/statistician who spent most of his life working at Berkeley University in the USA. He made a number of major contributions to the field of statistics, including introducing the concept of confidence intervals (see Chapter 4) and some foundational work on hypothe-

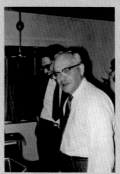
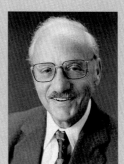

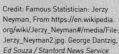
Credit: Famous Statistician: Jerzy Neyman, From https://en.wikipedia. org/wiki/Jerzy_Neyman#/media/File: Jerzy_Neyman2.jpg. George Dantzig, *Ed Souza / Stanford News Service*

sis testing (see Chapter 5). Dantzig was born in 1914 to Russian immigrants in the USA. Dantzig initially studied mathematics but gave it up because of his distaste for its "abstractness". He got a job as a statistician and then went to work for the famous statistician Jerzy Neyman at Berkeley. The rest of their story is told in Dantzig's own words:

"During my first year at Berkeley I arrived late one day to one of Neyman's classes. On the blackboard were two problems which I assumed had been assigned for homework. I copied them down. A few days later I apologized to Neyman for taking so long to do the homework – the problems seemed to be a little harder to do than usual. I asked him if he still wanted the work. He told me to throw it on his desk. I did so reluctantly because his desk was covered with such a heap of papers that I feared my homework would be lost there forever. About six weeks later, one Sunday morning about eight o'clock, Anne and I were awakened by someone banging on our front door. It was Neyman. He rushed in with papers in hand, all excited: 'I've just written an introduction to one of your papers. Read it so I can send it out right away for publication.' For a minute, I had no idea what he was talking about. To make a long story short, the problems on the blackboard which I had solved thinking they were homework were in fact two famous unsolved problems in statistics. That was the first inkling I had that there was anything special about them."

One of these problems was to provide a mathematical basis for Gosset's t-function (see Chapter 5). Neyman took the initiative in getting Dantzig's papers published and thus in launching Dantzig's career, which was long and active. Therefore, as well as a distinguished career of his own, Jerzy Neyman can take some credit for the contributions of George Dantzig. Neyman died in 1981 aged 81 in California. Dantzig died in 2005 aged 90, also in California.

CHAPTER 11

MATLAB Case Study on Descriptive and Inferential Statistics

11.1   INTRODUCTION

This chapter is slightly different to the others in this book. We do not attempt to introduce any new statistical concepts or techniques. Rather, we aim to illustrate how the concepts and techniques that we have learnt in this book can be applied to a real-world biomedical problem. Therefore, this is the only chapter of the book that requires competency in MATLAB and access to a computer running MATLAB. If you are not interested in the use of MATLAB for statistical analysis, you are advised to skip this chapter.

First, we introduce the motivation for the case study. The *left ventricle* is the chamber of the heart that pumps oxygenated blood into the aorta and round the body. The *myocardium* is the muscle that encloses the ventricle and provides the pumping action. There is significant clinical interest in measuring the thickness of the left ventricular myocardium. For example, such measurements can be useful for detecting infarcted regions (i.e. necrotic tissue as a result of reduced blood supply) or for diagnosing or studying the mechanisms of heart disease. Imaging offers an attractive noninvasive means to make these measurements.

In this case study, you will perform statistical analysis on myocardium thicknesses measured from magnetic resonance (MR) images. You will be provided with a number of MR slices of hearts of different subjects. You will use MATLAB to make measurements of myocardium thickness and then perform some statistical analysis on the resulting thickness data.

229

Statistics for Biomedical Engineers and Scientists. https://doi.org/10.1016/B978-0-08-102939-8.00020-7

11.2 DATA

The data used are the same MR data that the points used in Chapter 10 were derived from. The data set consists of 20 MR slices of human left ventricles, and these images are available to you from the web site of the book. You should first download these images and store them locally on your computer.

11.3 PART A: MEASURING MYOCARDIUM THICKNESS

The first task is to write code to enable a user to make interactive measurements of myocardial thickness from the images.

■ **Activity 11.1**

O11.A   Use MATLAB to perform the following tasks:

1. Write a function that takes a single image as its only argument, displays this image, allows the user to select two points by mouse clicking, and then returns as a result the distance between these two points. *The distance should be in millimeters, not pixels.* To convert from pixels to millimeters you will need the information that the 128×128 image arrays represent a physical field of view of 160×160 mm.

2. Write code to read all 20 images into a single three-dimensional array, i.e. each image is a 128×128 image, so the final array should be $128 \times 128 \times 20$. Then, for each image in the array, call your function to interactively measure the myocardium thickness of the image. Store these thicknesses in another array.

3. Modify the code so that it allows the user to make the set of measurements several times and stores them in a 2D array. For example, if you make 5 sets of measurements from the 20 images, the result should be a 5×20 array of measurements.

■

The following MATLAB function may be useful to you in completing this part of the case study (see the MATLAB documentation for more detail).

■ `[x,y] = ginput(n)`. Allows the user to select n points in the current figure by mouse clicking and stores the resulting coordinates (in pixels) of the points in the arrays x and y.

Once your code is complete and you are satisfied that it is working correctly, use it to measure the *maximum* myocardium thickness for each image in the data set, that is, decide at which point the myocardium is at its thickest and click on one point on the inner boundary and one point on the outer bound-

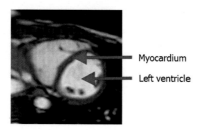

FIGURE 11.1
A cardiac MR slice annotated to show the myocardium, which is the dark area surrounding the left ventricle.

ary. Fig. 11.1 shows a sample image annotated to indicate the myocardium. Make several such measurements for each image.

11.4   PART B: INTRAOBSERVER VARIABILITY

In this part of the case study, you will analyze the measurement data to assess the *intraobserver* variability in measuring the myocardium thicknesses. In other words, what is the variation in the different measurements that you have made? A related concept is the *interobserver variability*, which refers to the variation in measurements made by *different* observers.

■ Activity 11.2

Use MATLAB to perform the following tasks: *O11.A*

1. Plot a histogram for each of the 20 images indicating the spread of measurements of myocardium thickness. Do they look symmetrically distributed? Do they look normally distributed?
2. Based on your answers, choose and compute appropriate measures of central tendency and variation to summarize the myocardium thickness data. You should compute these measures separately for each image but use the same measures for all images.

The measure of variation indicates the intraobserver variability in measuring the myocardium thicknesses. What do you think could cause this variability? How could the experiment be designed to minimize it?   ■

11.5   PART C: SAMPLE ANALYSIS

Now we will analyze this sample of measurements and compare it to another set of measurements for a different patient cohort. Use the central tendency values of your measurements as the first data set. The data for the new patient cohort is contained in the file "myo_data_cohort2.mat". Download this file from the book's web site and use it as the second data set.

We want to perform an appropriate statistical test to see if the two sets of data (the original and the new cohort arrays) are samples from the same distribution or not. To choose an appropriate test, we first need to know if the two data sets are normally distributed. In Chapter 7, we saw several visual and numerical techniques that can be used to determine if a sample was drawn from a normal distribution.

■ Activity 11.3

O11.A   Use MATLAB to perform the following tasks:

1. Use appropriate techniques and tests to determine if either/both of the two data sets are normally distributed.
2. Based on your findings about the distributions of the two data sets and on the type of data that they represent, choose an appropriate statistical test to decide if there is a significant difference between the myocardium thickness measurements of the two cohorts.
■

11.6   SUMMARY

This chapter has provided an example case study on statistical analysis of biomedical engineering data. It is often difficult to acquire data for statistical analysis, and in the real world, careful attention should be paid to experimental design. The amount of data available is often limited due to ethical and cost restrictions, and data processing methods need to be carefully designed to obtain the maximum amount of information from the available data, for example, minimizing or at the least quantifying intraobserver and/or interobserver variation if the measurements are to be made manually. Such considerations can pay dividends later in the project if more powerful statistical tools can be applied to infer conclusions.

FAMOUS STATISTICIAN: FLORENCE NIGHTINGALE DAVID

Florence Nightingale David was born in 1909 and was a renowned English statistician. She was named after Florence Nightingale (the famous founder of the modern nursing profession), who was a friend of her parents. Florence (the statistician) studied mathematics, then worked for Karl Pearson (see Chapter 1's Famous Statistician) at University College London. After Karl Pearson died in 1936, she went to work with Jerzy Neyman (see Chapter 10's Famous Statistician), where she submitted her last four published papers as her PhD thesis.

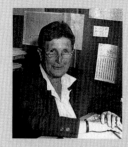

Credit: Famous Statistician: Florence Nightingale David, From Nan M. Laird, A Conversation with F. N. David, Statistical Science 1989, Vol. 4, No. 3, 235–246, http://www.dcscience.net/conversation-with-Florence-Nightingale-David.pdf

During World War II, Florence worked in the UK for the Ministry of Home Security. In late 1939 when war had started but England had not yet been attacked, she created statistical models to predict the possible consequences of bombs exploding in high-density populations such as the big cities of England and especially London. From these models she determined estimates of harm to humans and damage to nonhumans. This included the possible numbers living and dead, the reactions to fires, damaged buildings as well as damage to communications, and utilities such as phones, water, gas, electricity, and sewers. As a result, when London was bombed in 1940 and 1941, vital services were kept going, and her models were updated and modified with the evidence from the real harm and real damage. Florence died aged 83 in 1995 in Hertfordshire, UK.

Statistical Tables

Table A.1 Critical Student's t-test values (2-tailed) for significance levels 0.1, 0.05, and 0.01. Double the significance level for a 1-tailed test.

Degrees of freedom	Significance level 0.10	0.05	0.01	Degrees of freedom	Significance level 0.10	0.05	0.01
1	6.314	12.706	63.657	19	1.729	2.093	2.861
2	2.920	4.303	9.925	20	1.725	2.086	2.845
3	2.353	3.182	5.841	21	1.721	2.080	2.831
4	2.132	2.776	4.604	22	1.717	2.074	2.819
5	2.015	2.571	4.032	23	1.714	2.069	2.807
6	1.943	2.447	3.707	24	1.711	2.064	2.797
7	1.895	2.365	3.499	25	1.708	2.060	2.787
8	1.860	2.306	3.355	26	1.706	2.056	2.779
9	1.833	2.262	3.250	27	1.703	2.052	2.771
10	1.812	2.228	3.169	28	1.701	2.048	2.763
11	1.796	2.201	3.106	29	1.699	2.045	2.756
12	1.782	2.179	3.055	30	1.697	2.042	2.750
13	1.771	2.160	3.012	31	1.695	2.040	2.744
14	1.761	2.145	2.977	32	1.694	2.037	2.738
15	1.753	2.131	2.947	33	1.692	2.035	2.733
16	1.746	2.120	2.921	34	1.691	2.032	2.728
17	1.740	2.110	2.898	35	1.690	2.030	2.724
18	1.734	2.101	2.878	36	1.688	2.028	2.719

Table A.2 Critical z-test values (2-tailed) for significance levels 0.1, 0.05, 0.02, and 0.01. Double the significance level for a 1-tailed test.

	Significance level			
	0.1	**0.05**	**0.02**	**0.01**
Critical values:	1.65	1.96	2.33	2.58

Table A.3 Wilcoxon signed rank test critical values.

Level of significance for 1-tailed test				
	0.05	**0.025**	**0.01**	**0.005**
Level of significance for 2-tailed test				
n	**0.1**	**0.05**	**0.02**	**0.01**
5	0			
6	2	0		
7	3	2	0	
8	5	3	1	0
9	8	5	3	1
10	10	8	5	3
11	13	10	7	5
12	17	13	9	7
13	21	17	12	9
14	25	21	15	12
15	30	25	19	15
16	35	29	23	19
17	41	34	27	23
18	47	40	32	27
19	53	46	37	32
20	60	52	43	37
21	67	58	49	42
22	75	65	55	48
23	83	73	62	54
24	91	81	69	61
25	100	89	76	68

Table A.4 Mann–Whitney U test critical values, 2-tailed test, 0.05 significance level. This table can also be used for a 1-tailed test at 0.025 significance level.

n_c	n_t											
	1	2	3	4	5	6	7	8	9	10	11	12
1	–	–	–	–	–	–	–	–	–	–	–	–
2	–	–	–	–	–	–	–	0	0	0	0	1
3	–	–	–	–	0	1	1	2	2	3	3	4
4	–	–	–	0	1	2	3	4	4	5	6	7
5	–	–	0	1	2	3	5	6	7	8	9	11
6	–	–	1	2	3	5	6	8	10	11	13	14
7	–	–	1	3	5	6	8	10	12	14	16	18
8	–	0	2	4	6	8	10	13	15	17	19	22
9	–	0	2	4	7	10	12	15	17	20	23	26
10	–	0	3	5	8	11	14	17	20	23	26	29
11	–	0	3	6	9	13	16	19	23	26	30	33
12	–	1	4	7	11	14	18	22	26	29	33	37

Table A.5 Critical values of χ^2 test with v degrees of freedom and significance levels of 0.05, 0.025, and 0.01.

v	Significance level		
	0.05	0.025	0.01
1	3.841	5.024	6.635
2	5.991	7.378	9.210
3	7.815	9.348	11.345
4	9.488	11.143	13.277
5	11.070	12.833	15.086
6	12.592	14.449	16.812
7	14.067	16.013	18.475
8	15.507	17.535	20.090
9	16.919	19.023	21.666
10	18.307	20.483	23.209
11	19.675	21.920	24.725
12	21.026	23.337	26.217
13	22.362	24.736	27.688
14	23.685	26.119	29.141
15	24.996	27.488	30.578
16	26.296	28.845	32.000
17	27.587	30.191	33.409
18	28.869	31.526	34.805
19	30.144	32.852	36.191
20	31.410	34.170	37.566
21	32.671	35.479	38.932
22	33.924	36.781	40.289
23	35.172	38.076	41.638
24	36.415	39.364	42.980
25	37.652	40.646	44.314
26	38.885	41.923	45.642
27	40.113	43.195	46.963
28	41.337	44.461	48.278
29	42.557	45.722	49.588
30	43.773	46.979	50.892

Table A.6 Coefficients for the Shapiro–Wilk test for normality (for $n \leq 25$).

$n =$	2	3	4	5	6	7	8	9	10	11	12	13
a_1	0.7071	0.7071	0.6872	0.6646	0.6431	0.6233	0.6052	0.5888	0.5739	0.5601	0.5475	0.5359
a_2		0.0	0.1677	0.2143	0.2806	0.3031	0.3164	0.3244	0.3291	0.3315	0.3325	0.3325
a_3				0.0	0.0875	0.1401	0.1743	0.1976	0.2141	0.226	0.2347	0.2412
a_4						0.0	0.0561	0.0947	0.1224	0.1429	0.1586	0.1707
a_5								0.0	0.0399	0.0695	0.0922	0.1099
a_6										0.0	0.0303	0.0539
a_7												0.0

$n =$	14	15	16	17	18	19	20	21	22	23	24	25
a_1	0.5251	0.515	0.5056	0.4968	0.4886	0.4808	0.4734	0.4643	0.459	0.4542	0.4493	0.445
a_2	0.3318	0.3306	0.329	0.3273	0.3253	0.3232	0.3211	0.3185	0.3156	0.3126	0.3098	0.3069
a_3	0.246	0.2495	0.2521	0.254	0.2553	0.2561	0.2565	0.2578	0.2571	0.2563	0.2554	0.2543
a_4	0.1802	0.1878	0.1939	0.1988	0.2027	0.2059	0.2085	0.2119	0.2131	0.2139	0.2145	0.2148
a_5	0.124	0.1353	0.1447	0.1524	0.1587	0.1641	0.1686	0.1736	0.1764	0.1787	0.1807	0.1822
a_6	0.0727	0.088	0.1005	0.1109	0.1197	0.1271	0.1334	0.1399	0.1443	0.148	0.1512	0.1539
a_7	0.024	0.0433	0.0593	0.0725	0.0837	0.0932	0.1013	0.1092	0.115	0.1201	0.1245	0.1283
a_8		0.0	0.0196	0.0359	0.0496	0.0612	0.0711	0.0804	0.0878	0.0941	0.0997	0.1046
a_9				0.0	0.0163	0.0303	0.0422	0.053	0.0618	0.0696	0.0764	0.0823
a_{10}						0.0	0.014	0.0263	0.0368	0.0459	0.0539	0.061
a_{11}								0.0	0.0122	0.0228	0.0321	0.0403
a_{12}										0.0	0.0107	0.02
a_{13}												0.0

Table A.7 Shapiro–Wilk test critical values of *Tab W.*

Level of significance				
n	**0.01**	**0.02**	**0.05**	**0.1**
3	0.753	0.756	0.767	0.789
4	0.687	0.707	0.748	0.792
5	0.686	0.715	0.762	0.806
6	0.713	0.743	0.788	0.826
7	0.73	0.76	0.803	0.838
8	0.749	0.778	0.818	0.851
9	0.764	0.791	0.829	0.859
10	0.781	0.806	0.842	0.869
11	0.792	0.817	0.85	0.876
12	0.805	0.828	0.859	0.883
13	0.814	0.837	0.866	0.889
14	0.825	0.846	0.874	0.895
15	0.835	0.855	0.881	0.901
16	0.844	0.863	0.887	0.906
17	0.851	0.869	0.892	0.91
18	0.858	0.874	0.897	0.914
19	0.863	0.879	0.901	0.917
20	0.868	0.884	0.905	0.92
21	0.873	0.888	0.908	0.923
22	0.878	0.892	0.911	0.926
23	0.881	0.895	0.914	0.928
24	0.884	0.898	0.916	0.93
25	0.888	0.901	0.918	0.931

Table A.8 Critical values for the ANOVA F statistic at 0.05 significance: $k =$ number of groups, $N =$ total sample size (over all groups). Table shows values for MSE degrees of freedom from 1–50. See Table A.9 for 51–100.

MSE df: $N - k$	MSB degrees of freedom: $k - 1$									
	1	**2**	**3**	**4**	**5**	**6**	**7**	**8**	**9**	**10**
1	161.44	199.50	215.70	224.58	230.16	233.98	236.76	238.88	240.54	241.88
2	18.513	19.000	19.164	19.247	19.296	19.330	19.353	19.371	19.385	19.396
3	10.128	9.552	9.277	9.117	9.013	8.941	8.887	8.845	8.812	8.786
4	7.709	6.944	6.591	6.388	6.256	6.163	6.094	6.041	5.999	5.964
5	6.608	5.786	5.409	5.192	5.050	4.950	4.876	4.818	4.772	4.735
6	5.987	5.143	4.757	4.534	4.387	4.284	4.207	4.147	4.099	4.060
7	5.591	4.737	4.347	4.120	3.972	3.866	3.787	3.726	3.677	3.637
8	5.318	4.459	4.066	3.838	3.687	3.581	3.500	3.438	3.388	3.347
9	5.117	4.256	3.863	3.633	3.482	3.374	3.293	3.230	3.179	3.137
10	4.965	4.103	3.708	3.478	3.326	3.217	3.135	3.072	3.020	2.978
11	4.844	3.982	3.587	3.357	3.204	3.095	3.012	2.948	2.896	2.854
12	4.747	3.885	3.490	3.259	3.106	2.996	2.913	2.849	2.796	2.753
13	4.667	3.806	3.411	3.179	3.025	2.915	2.832	2.767	2.714	2.671
14	4.600	3.739	3.344	3.112	2.958	2.848	2.764	2.699	2.646	2.602
15	4.543	3.682	3.287	3.056	2.901	2.790	2.707	2.641	2.588	2.544
16	4.494	3.634	3.239	3.007	2.852	2.741	2.657	2.591	2.538	2.494
17	4.451	3.592	3.197	2.965	2.810	2.699	2.614	2.548	2.494	2.450
18	4.414	3.555	3.160	2.928	2.773	2.661	2.577	2.510	2.456	2.412
19	4.381	3.522	3.127	2.895	2.740	2.628	2.544	2.477	2.423	2.378
20	4.351	3.493	3.098	2.866	2.711	2.599	2.514	2.447	2.393	2.348
21	4.325	3.467	3.072	2.840	2.685	2.573	2.488	2.420	2.366	2.321
22	4.301	3.443	3.049	2.817	2.661	2.549	2.464	2.397	2.342	2.297
23	4.279	3.422	3.028	2.796	2.640	2.528	2.442	2.375	2.320	2.275
24	4.260	3.403	3.009	2.776	2.621	2.508	2.423	2.355	2.300	2.255
25	4.242	3.385	2.991	2.759	2.603	2.490	2.405	2.337	2.282	2.236
26	4.225	3.369	2.975	2.743	2.587	2.474	2.388	2.321	2.265	2.220
27	4.210	3.354	2.960	2.728	2.572	2.459	2.373	2.305	2.250	2.204
28	4.196	3.340	2.947	2.714	2.558	2.445	2.359	2.291	2.236	2.190
29	4.183	3.328	2.934	2.701	2.545	2.432	2.346	2.278	2.223	2.177
30	4.171	3.316	2.922	2.690	2.534	2.421	2.334	2.266	2.211	2.165
31	4.160	3.305	2.911	2.679	2.523	2.409	2.323	2.255	2.199	2.153
32	4.149	3.295	2.901	2.668	2.512	2.399	2.313	2.244	2.189	2.142
33	4.139	3.285	2.892	2.659	2.503	2.389	2.303	2.235	2.179	2.133
34	4.130	3.276	2.883	2.650	2.494	2.380	2.294	2.225	2.170	2.123
35	4.121	3.267	2.874	2.641	2.485	2.372	2.285	2.217	2.161	2.114

(continued on next page)

Table A.8 (*continued*)

MSE df: $N - k$	MSB degrees of freedom: $k - 1$									
	1	**2**	**3**	**4**	**5**	**6**	**7**	**8**	**9**	**10**
36	4.113	3.259	2.866	2.634	2.477	2.364	2.277	2.209	2.153	2.106
37	4.105	3.252	2.859	2.626	2.470	2.356	2.270	2.201	2.145	2.098
38	4.098	3.245	2.852	2.619	2.463	2.349	2.262	2.194	2.138	2.091
39	4.091	3.238	2.845	2.612	2.456	2.342	2.255	2.187	2.131	2.084
40	4.085	3.232	2.839	2.606	2.449	2.336	2.249	2.180	2.124	2.077
41	4.079	3.226	2.833	2.600	2.443	2.330	2.243	2.174	2.118	2.071
42	4.073	3.220	2.827	2.594	2.438	2.324	2.237	2.168	2.112	2.065
43	4.067	3.214	2.822	2.589	2.432	2.318	2.232	2.163	2.106	2.059
44	4.062	3.209	2.816	2.584	2.427	2.313	2.226	2.157	2.101	2.054
45	4.057	3.204	2.812	2.579	2.422	2.308	2.221	2.152	2.096	2.049
46	4.052	3.200	2.807	2.574	2.417	2.304	2.216	2.147	2.091	2.044
47	4.047	3.195	2.802	2.570	2.413	2.299	2.212	2.143	2.086	2.039
48	4.043	3.191	2.798	2.565	2.409	2.295	2.207	2.138	2.082	2.035
49	4.038	3.187	2.794	2.561	2.404	2.290	2.203	2.134	2.077	2.030
50	4.034	3.183	2.790	2.557	2.400	2.286	2.199	2.130	2.073	2.026

Table A.9 Critical values for the ANOVA F statistic at 0.05 significance: $k = $ number of groups, $N = $ total sample size (over all groups). Table shows values for MSE degrees of freedom from 51–100. See Table A.8 for 1–50.

MSE df: $N - k$	MSB degrees of freedom: $k - 1$									
	1	**2**	**3**	**4**	**5**	**6**	**7**	**8**	**9**	**10**
51	4.030	3.179	2.786	2.553	2.397	2.283	2.195	2.126	2.069	2.022
52	4.027	3.175	2.783	2.550	2.393	2.279	2.192	2.122	2.066	2.018
53	4.023	3.172	2.779	2.546	2.389	2.275	2.188	2.119	2.062	2.015
54	4.020	3.168	2.776	2.543	2.386	2.272	2.185	2.115	2.059	2.011
55	4.016	3.165	2.773	2.540	2.383	2.269	2.181	2.112	2.055	2.008
56	4.013	3.162	2.769	2.537	2.380	2.266	2.178	2.109	2.052	2.005
57	4.010	3.159	2.766	2.534	2.377	2.263	2.175	2.106	2.049	2.001
58	4.007	3.156	2.764	2.531	2.374	2.260	2.172	2.103	2.046	1.998
59	4.004	3.153	2.761	2.528	2.371	2.257	2.169	2.100	2.043	1.995
60	4.001	3.150	2.758	2.525	2.368	2.254	2.167	2.097	2.040	1.993
61	3.998	3.148	2.755	2.523	2.366	2.251	2.164	2.094	2.037	1.990
62	3.996	3.145	2.753	2.520	2.363	2.249	2.161	2.092	2.035	1.987
63	3.993	3.143	2.751	2.518	2.361	2.246	2.159	2.089	2.032	1.985
64	3.991	3.140	2.748	2.515	2.358	2.244	2.156	2.087	2.030	1.982

(continued on next page)

Table A.9 (*continued*)

MSE df:	MSB degrees of freedom: $k - 1$									
$N - k$	1	2	3	4	5	6	7	8	9	10
65	3.989	3.138	2.746	2.513	2.356	2.242	2.154	2.084	2.027	1.980
66	3.986	3.136	2.744	2.511	2.354	2.239	2.152	2.082	2.025	1.977
67	3.984	3.134	2.742	2.509	2.352	2.237	2.150	2.080	2.023	1.975
68	3.982	3.132	2.740	2.507	2.350	2.235	2.148	2.078	2.021	1.973
69	3.980	3.130	2.737	2.505	2.348	2.233	2.145	2.076	2.019	1.971
70	3.978	3.128	2.736	2.503	2.346	2.231	2.143	2.074	2.017	1.969
71	3.976	3.126	2.734	2.501	2.344	2.229	2.142	2.072	2.015	1.967
72	3.974	3.124	2.732	2.499	2.342	2.227	2.140	2.070	2.013	1.965
73	3.972	3.122	2.730	2.497	2.340	2.226	2.138	2.068	2.011	1.963
74	3.970	3.120	2.728	2.495	2.338	2.224	2.136	2.066	2.009	1.961
75	3.968	3.119	2.727	2.494	2.337	2.222	2.134	2.064	2.007	1.959
76	3.967	3.117	2.725	2.492	2.335	2.220	2.133	2.063	2.006	1.958
77	3.965	3.115	2.723	2.490	2.333	2.219	2.131	2.061	2.004	1.956
78	3.963	3.114	2.722	2.489	2.332	2.217	2.129	2.059	2.002	1.954
79	3.962	3.112	2.720	2.487	2.330	2.216	2.128	2.058	2.001	1.953
80	3.960	3.111	2.719	2.486	2.329	2.214	2.126	2.056	1.999	1.951
81	3.959	3.109	2.717	2.484	2.327	2.213	2.125	2.055	1.998	1.950
82	3.957	3.108	2.716	2.483	2.326	2.211	2.123	2.053	1.996	1.948
83	3.956	3.107	2.715	2.482	2.324	2.210	2.122	2.052	1.995	1.947
84	3.955	3.105	2.713	2.480	2.323	2.209	2.121	2.051	1.993	1.945
85	3.953	3.104	2.712	2.479	2.322	2.207	2.119	2.049	1.992	1.944
86	3.952	3.103	2.711	2.478	2.321	2.206	2.118	2.048	1.991	1.943
87	3.951	3.101	2.709	2.476	2.319	2.205	2.117	2.047	1.989	1.941
88	3.949	3.100	2.708	2.475	2.318	2.203	2.115	2.045	1.988	1.940
89	3.948	3.099	2.707	2.474	2.317	2.202	2.114	2.044	1.987	1.939
90	3.947	3.098	2.706	2.473	2.316	2.201	2.113	2.043	1.986	1.938
91	3.946	3.097	2.705	2.472	2.315	2.200	2.112	2.042	1.984	1.936
92	3.945	3.095	2.704	2.471	2.313	2.199	2.111	2.041	1.983	1.935
93	3.943	3.094	2.703	2.470	2.312	2.198	2.110	2.040	1.982	1.934
94	3.942	3.093	2.701	2.469	2.311	2.197	2.109	2.038	1.981	1.933
95	3.941	3.092	2.700	2.467	2.310	2.196	2.108	2.037	1.980	1.932
96	3.940	3.091	2.699	2.466	2.309	2.195	2.106	2.036	1.979	1.931
97	3.939	3.090	2.698	2.465	2.308	2.194	2.105	2.035	1.978	1.930
98	3.938	3.089	2.697	2.465	2.307	2.193	2.104	2.034	1.977	1.929
99	3.937	3.088	2.696	2.464	2.306	2.192	2.103	2.033	1.976	1.928
100	3.936	3.087	2.696	2.463	2.305	2.191	2.103	2.032	1.975	1.927

References

1. S. Cohen, D. Janicki-Deverts, Who's stressed? Distributions of psychological stress in the United States in probability samples from 1983, 2006, and 2009, Journal of Applied Psychology 42 (6) (2012) 1320–1334.

2. D.G. Altman, J.M. Bland, Measurement in medicine: The analysis of method comparison studies, Journal of the Royal Statistical Society. Series D (The Statistician) 32 (3) (1983) 307–317.

3. D. Giavarina, Understanding Bland Altman analysis, Biochemia Medica 25 (2) (2015) 141–151.

4. W. Casscells, A. Schoenberger, T. Grayboys, Interpretation by physicians of clinical laboratory results, New England Journal of Medicine 18 (1978) 999–1001.

5. M. Zweig, G. Campbell, Receiver operating characteristics (ROC) plots: A fundamental evaluation tool in clinical medicine, Clinical Chemistry 39 (4) (1993) 561–577.

6. H. Mann, D.R. Whitney, On a test of whether one of two random variables is stochastically larger than the other, Annals of Mathematical Statistics 18 (1947) 50–60.

7. T.J. Scanlon, R.N. Luben, F.L. Scanlon, N. Singleton, Is Friday the 13th bad for your health?, British Medical Journal 307 (6919) (1993) 1584–1586.

8. H. Hotelling, The generalization of student's ratio, Annals of Mathematical Statistics 2 (3) (1931) 360–378.

9. T.F. Cootes, C.J. Taylor, D.H. Cooper, J. Graham, Active shape models – their training and application, Computer Vision and Image Understanding 61 (1) (1995) 38–59.

10. O. Ecabert, J. Peters, H. Schramm, C. Lorenz, J. von Berg, M.J. Walker, M. Vembar, M.E. Olszewski, K. Subramanyan, G. Lavi, J. Weese, Automatic model-based segmentation of the heart in CT images, IEEE Transactions on Medical Imaging 27 (9) (2008) 1189–1201.

11. T. Heimann, H.P. Meinzer, Statistical shape models for 3D medical image segmentation: A review, Medical Image Analysis 13 (4) (2009) 543–563.

12. P.A. Yushkevich, J. Piven, H.C. Hazlett, R.G. Smith, S. Ho, J.C. Gee, G. Gerig, User-guided 3D active contour segmentation of anatomical structures: significantly improved efficiency and reliability, Neuroimage 31 (3) (2006) 1116–1128.

13. J.R. McClelland, D.J. Hawkes, T. Schaeffter, A.P. King, Respiratory motion models: A review, Medical Image Analysis 17 (2013) 19–42.

14. N. Duchateau, M.D. Craene, G. Piella, E. Silva, A. Doltra, M. Sitges, B.H. Bijnens, A.F. Frangi, A spatiotemporal statistical atlas of motion for the quantification of abnormal myocardial tissue velocities, Medical Image Analysis 15 (3) (2011) 316–328.

Index